AF327022

Progress in Hepatology, Volume 4
Liver Cirrhosis Update

Progress in Hepatology, Volume 4
Liver Cirrhosis Update

Proceedings of the 'Takahashi Memorial Forum', held in Tokyo, Japan, on 15 November 1997

Editors:

Masami Yamanaka
Department of Medicine
Teikyo University School of Medicine
Tokyo, Japan

Gotaro Toda
Department of Internal Medicine (I)
Jikei University School of Medicine
Tokyo, Japan

Teruji Tanaka
Department of Internal Medicine (I)
Jikei University School of Medicine, Daisan Hospital
Tokyo, Japan

Associate Editors:

Mikio Zeniya
Department of Internal Medicine (I)
Jikei University School of Medicine
Tokyo, Japan

Hajime Takikawa
Department of Medicine
Teikyo University School of Medicine
Tokyo, Japan

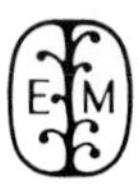

1998

ELSEVIER

Amsterdam – Lausanne – New York – Oxford – Shannon – Singapore – Tokyo

ELSEVIER SCIENCE B.V.
Sara Burgerhartstraat 25
P.O. Box 211, 1000 AE Amsterdam, The Netherlands

First edition 1998

Library of Congress Cataloging in Publication Data
A catalog record from the Library of Congress has been applied for.

International Congress Series No. 1163
ISBN: 0 444 82940 7

Printed in the Netherlands

Preface

This volume of *Progress in Hepatology* includes the basic and clinical research on liver cirrhosis and its treatment. This was presented at the fourth Tadao Takahashi Memorial Forum held in Tokyo in 1997.

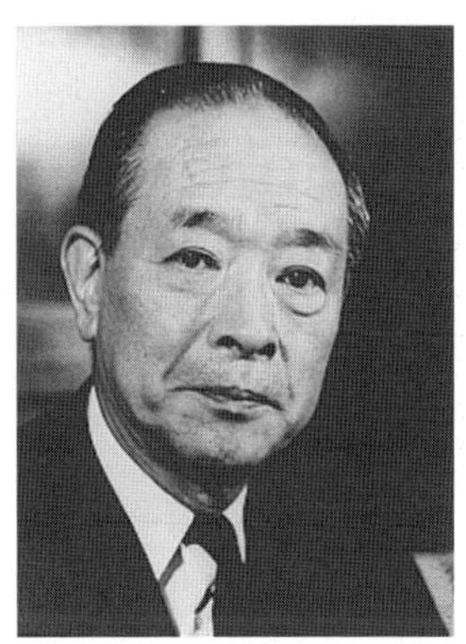

Liver cirrhosis is a final outcome of almost all chronic liver diseases. The etiology differs markedly among various countries. In Japan, and probably in the countries of East and South-East Asia, hepatitis B virus and/or hepatitis C virus are the most common cause of liver cirrhosis. In western countries, however, alcohol is the most common cause. In Japan, alcohol-induced liver cirrhosis was found in only 10% of those classified on the etiological basis in a nationwide survey conducted in 1991. Cirrhosis is the result of continuing hepatocellular injury followed by fibrosis and regeneration. The mechanism of hepatocyte injury differed between virus- and alcohol-induced chronic liver diseases. In the former, there have been several lines of evidence indicating that immunological attack against virus-infected hepatocyte plays a role in the perpetuation of hepatocyte injury; in the latter, alcohol and its metabolite produced within the hepatocyte is important in the development and perpetuation of hepatocyte injury; also malnutrition, which is often associated with alcoholic abuse, may potentiate the deleterious effect. These differences will produce pathological, functional and, more importantly, clinical features of etiologically different liver cirrhosis, the final outcome of continuing hepatocellular injury. One of the most important differences is the high frequency of development of hepatocellular carcinoma in virus-induced cirrhotic liver. In Japan, patients with liver cirrhosis used to die of variceral bleeding and hepatic failure without hepatocellular carcinoma. Recently, very few patients have died without hepatocellular carcinoma. This is probably due to advances in nutritional therapy and the treatment of major complications of liver cirrhosis. Even in the patients with hepatocellular carcinoma, however, the treatment of liver cirrhosis is important, because about 80% or more of the patients with hepatocellular carcinoma have liver cirrhosis.

In this volume of *Progress in Hepatology*, the present status of basic and clinical research on liver cirrhosis and its treatment in Japan is presented. Liver cirrhosis discussed in each chapter is almost exclusively due to HCV and/or HBV. We hope that this volume helps the readers to know the present status of liver cirrhosis and its treatment in Japan, where the main cause of liver cirrhosis is hepatitis viruses.

Gotaro Toda, MD
Professor of Department of Internal Medicine (1)
The Jikei University School of Medicine

Contents

Progress in Hepatology, Volume 4.
Liver Cirrhosis Update.
M. Yamanaka et al., editors.

Classification of liver cirrhosis in Japan: a pathological aspect

Masahiko Okudaira

Kitasato University, Kitasto; and Department of Pathology, Japan Bioassay Research Center, Japan Industrial Health and Safety Association, Kanagawa, Japan

Abstract. Liver cirrhosis is one of the most common diseases in Japan, with an incidence of almost 7% among the Japanese pathological autopsy cases. Nagayo-Miyake's classification for common types of liver cirrhosis has been widely used in Japan not only by a majority of pathologists but also by many clinicians. Morbid anatomical findings of Nagayo-Miyake's type A (postnecrotic) cirrhosis, type A′ (advanced stage of type A and type B), type B (posthepatitic), type B′ (precirrhotic stage of type B), and type F (alcoholic) cirrhosis are briefly documented. Representative intrahepatic vascular alterations are shown, and a peculiar feature of a nonhyalinized stromal connective tissue in cirrhotic livers are also demonstrated. The concept of pseudohypertrophic cirrhosis for denoting alcoholic hypertrophic cirrhosis is also mentioned. It is my hope that liver cirrhosis will become a curable disease in the coming 21st century.

Keywords: morbid anatomical features, Nagayo-Miyake's classification, pseudohypertrophic cirrhosis, pseudonodule, vascular alterations.

Introduction

Although it has been stated that the cirrhotic change of the liver had been recognized by Greeks and Romans long before [1] the term "liver cirrhosis" had been introduced in the medical literature by Laennec (1826) [2]. This was the Tokugawa era of the 11th Shogun Ienari Tokugawa, and Chinese medicine was popular in Japan. However, western medicine was unfamiliar and thought to know almost nothing about liver cirrhosis.

The first authentic morbid anatomical research on liver cirrhosis was reported by Nagayo at the 4th Annual Congress of the Japanese Pathological Society (1915) [3]. Since then, Nagayo's classification of liver cirrhosis has been widely used in Japan, not only by pathologists but also by clinicians.

At the present time, liver cirrhosis is a common disease in Japan: the number of deaths caused by the disease reached almost 17,000 in 1992 [4], ranking eighth in the order of main causes of death in vital statistics.

Among Japanese pathological autopsy cases, the incidence of liver cirrhosis is almost 7%, the male to female ratio is 7:3, and a peak aging incidence is found in the fifth to seventh decades. Geographically, many more cases have been encountered in south-western regions than in north-eastern regions [5].

Address for correspondence: Masahiko Okudaira MD, PhD, Head, Department of Pathology, Japan Bioassay Research Center, Japan Industrial Health and Safety Association, 2445 Hirasawa, Hadano, Kanagawa 257-0015, Japan.

Definition and morphological findings of liver cirrhosis

In 1965, a morphologic criteria of liver cirrhosis was proposed by the research committee on liver cirrhosis, aided a by grant from The Japanese Ministry of Education [6]. The criteria consisted of the following four points:
1) macroscopical nodule formation;
2) connective tissue septa formation between portal areas and central veins and/ or hepatic veins;
3) architectural distortion of hepatic lobules; and
4) diffuse change in the entire liver.
These criteria could be simplified by saying that liver cirrhosis is a pathological condition with diffuse pseudonodule formations in the entire liver.

The term "pseudonodule" is synonymous with regenerated nodule and/or disorganized or distorted hepatic lobule, and is defined as a macroscopically identifiable nodular mass of hepatocytes that is surrounded by connective tissue septa. Pseudolobules lose normal topographical relations between portal tracts and terminal hepatic venules. It should be realized that haptic architectural distortions in and around pseudolobules are recognizable without exception, not only in the hepatic parenchyma but also in stromal connective tissue, including hepatic vasculatures.

The principal processes in the development of liver cirrhosis are: 1) hepatic parenchymal destruction, 2) active proliferation of connective tissue, and 3) regeneration of hepatocytes in a distorted nodular fashion. The most fundamental hepatic change is a parenchymal destruction, and is, without exception, more prominent than hepatocytic regeneration. The proliferation of connective tissue could be assumed to be a reparative process for incomplete hepatocytic regeneration. Liver cirrhosis has been considered as an end stage lesion of chronic active liver diseases caused by hepatitis viruses, drugs, alcohol, autoimmune disease, and various other diseases. Moreover, most clinicians seem to assume, so far, that liver cirrhosis is an irreversible and terminal condition of liver diseases.

I have been investigating vascular changes in cirrhotic livers by injection study [7,8]. Some representative findings will be presented here.

Figure 1 shows conspicuous collateral circulatory routes in the chorda venae umbilicalis detected in a child case of postnecrotic liver cirrhosis. This shunt connects the intrahepatic portal vein and the subcutaneous vein of the abdominal wall.

Alterations of peripheral portal branches in cirrhotic livers have also been investigated. Barium mixed gelatin solution was injected into the portal vein of autopsy livers. After fixation, liver slices 1 to 2 cm in thickness were submitted for soft X-ray examination. Distortion of peripheral portal vein branches in micronodular cirrhosis is demonstrated in Fig. 2. Figure 3 illustrates a distorted pattern disclosed in a case of macronodular cirrhosis, and Fig. 4 indicates a marked alteration of portal vein branches found in megalonodular cirrhosis (Wilson's disease). It should be noticed that a distorted pattern of peripheral portal

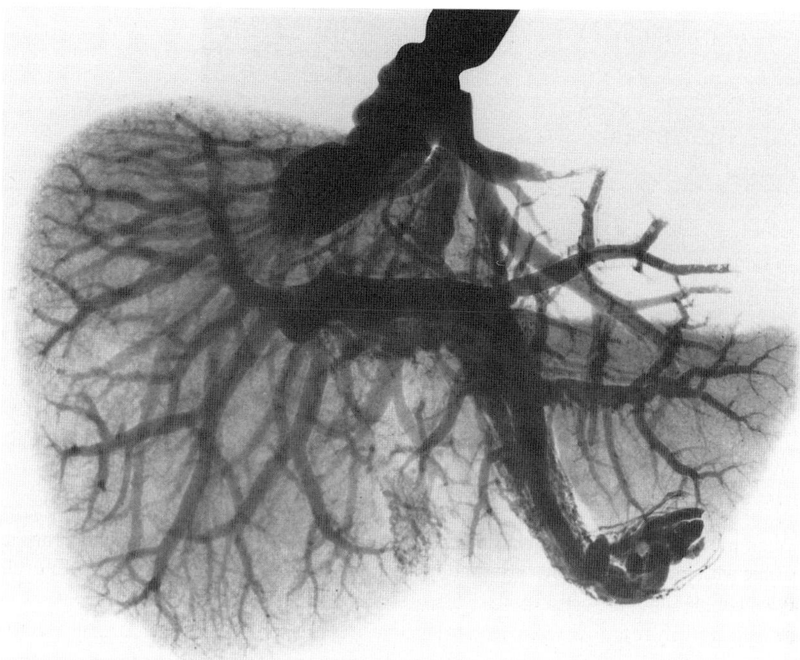

Fig. 1. Conspicuous collateral circulatory path was found in chorda venae umbilicalis in a child case with Nagayo-Miyake's type A cirrhosis. Soft X-ray photograph of plastic injected cast preparation. The collateral pathways consist chiefly of portal vein system and partly of hepatic artery system.

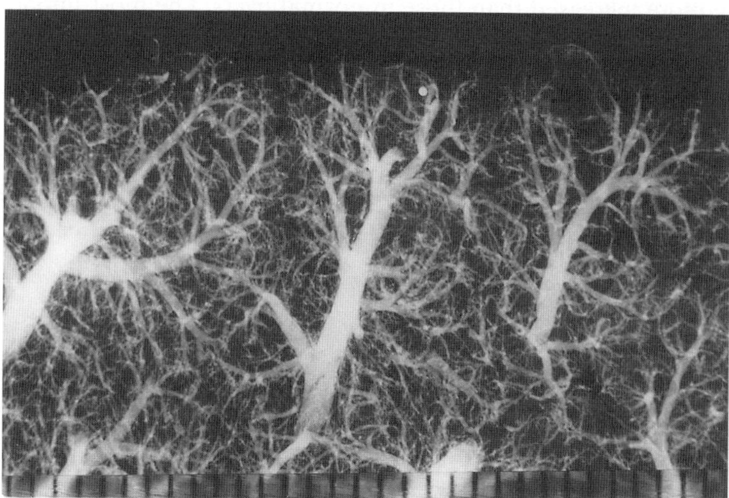

Fig. 2. Alteration of peripheral portal branches in a case with Miyake's type F cirrhosis, which is compatible with alcoholic cirrhosis. A Barium-mixed gelatin solution was injected into the portal vein of the autopsy case, and liver slices 1—2 cm in thickness were submitted for soft X-ray study. The scale on the bottom of the photograph is marked in mm.

4

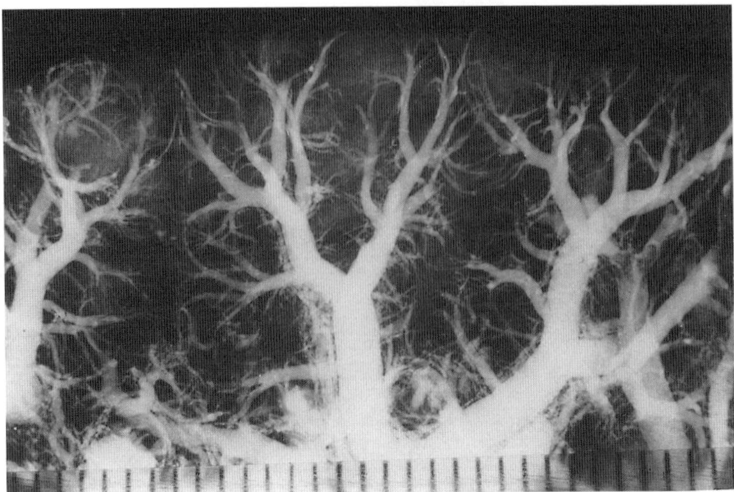

Fig. 3. Alteration of peripheral portal branches in a case with Nagayo-Miyake's type B liver cirrhosis, which is compatible with posthepatitic cirrhosis and macronodular cirrhosis. The distortion of portal veins is more conspicuous than those in Fig. 2.

branches was most prominent in a megalonodular cirrhosis, and was more marked in a macronodular cirrhosis than in a case with micronodular cirrhosis. Distortion of the peripheral portal branches and shunt formations were detected not only between hepatic arteries and portal veins and/or hepatic veins, but also between portal veins and hepatic veins. In most cases of liver cirrhosis, arterial vascular beds were more increased than those in normal livers. The most impor-

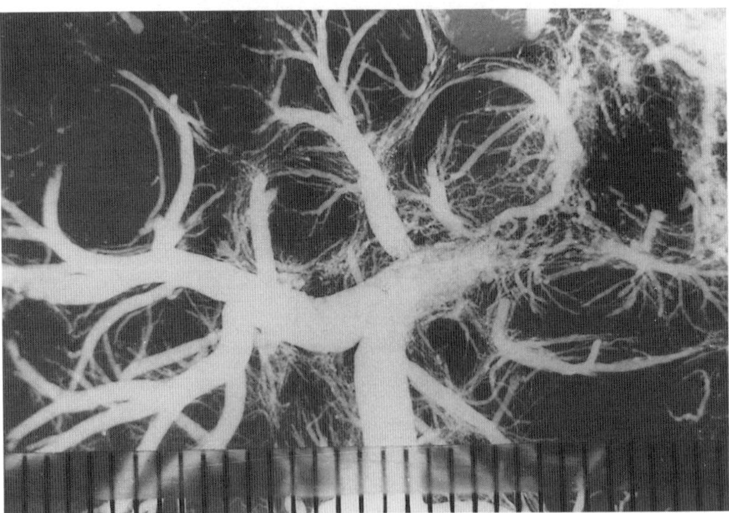

Fig. 4. Alteration of peripheral portal branches in a case with Wilson's disease (megalonodular cirrhosis). The distorted pattern of portal vein branches is most severe among those in Figs. 2—4.

tant hepatic microcirculatory disturbance in liver cirrhosis is reduced sinusoidal blood flow, and is incriminable for the functional disturbance of the liver. From this evidence, as Galambos [1] mentions, liver cirrhosis could be assumed to be a vascular disease.

Classification of liver cirrhosis in Japan

The most popular Japanese classification of liver cirrhosis [5,10] is shown in Table 1.

Nagayo's classification of atrophic liver cirrhosis was based not only on morbid anatomical findings and pathological sequelae but also on pathogenesis and clinical findings. Nagayo's type A and type B classification has been widely accepted in Japan, not only by pathologists but also by clinicians.

In 1960, Miyake [9] revised Nagayo's classification by adding the concept of the developmental stages of cirrhosis, and proposed A, A', B, and B' type classifications for atrophic cirrhosis.

Pathogenesis and morphologic characteristics of the three common types of cirrhosis in Japan are listed in Table 2.

Nagayo-Miyake's type A cirrhosis is compatible with postnecrotic type cirrhosis [5,10]. Macroscopically, the liver is reduced in size and increased in consistency. The entire liver is occupied by variously sized pseudolobules (macronodular and micronodular) with broad interstitial connective tissue (Figs. 5 and 6). Histopathologically, degenerative and necrotic changes of hepatocytes are prominent and abundant, inflammatory cell infiltrations composed chiefly of lymphocytes and plasma cells are noticed in broad connective tissue stroma. Marked bile ductular proliferation is also characteristic; however, no increase of elastic fibers is a constant feature. This type of cirrhosis is scarcely associated with hepatocellular carcinoma. A' type is an advanced stage of type A cirrhosis.

Nagayo-Miyake's type B liver cirrhosis is compatible with posthepatitic cirrhosis. This type of cirrhosis is a notorious sequela of chronic active hepatitis of viral origin. The precirrhotic stage of this type is called Miyake's type B' cirrhosis and is compatible with incomplete septal cirrhosis [11] (Fig. 7). Macroscopically, the B type cirrhosis is atrophic, and macronodular-pseudolobule formation with

Table 1. Morphological classification of liver cirrhosis in Japan.

Common type of liver cirrhosis
   1. Nagayo-Miyake's type A cirrhosis
   2. Nagayo-Miyake's type B cirrhosis
   3. Miyake's type F cirrhosis
Specific type of liver cirrhosis
   1. Congestive cirrhosis
   2. Biliary cirrhosis
   3. Parasitic cirrhosis
   4. Others (Wilson's disease, etc.)

6

Table 2. Pathogenesis and morphologic characteristics of three common types of cirrhosis in Japan.

	Nagayo-Miyake's type A cirrhosis	Nagayo-Miyake's type B cirrhosis	Miyake's type F cirrhosis
Etiology	Viral hepatitis, toxic injuries, etc.	Viral hepatitis, toxic injuries, etc.	Chronic alcoholism, malnutrition
Principal pathogenetic change	Massive hepatic necrosis	Chronic hepatitis	Longstanding and severe fatty liver
Precirrhotic stage[a]	Subacute liver atrophy	Miyake's type B′ cirrhosis (incomplete hepatic cirrhosis)	Fatty liver with fibrosis
Completed stage[a]	(Postnecrotic cirrhosis)	(Posthepatic cirrhosis)	(Alcoholic cirrhosis)
Advanced stage	Miyake's type A′ cirrhosis	Miyake's type A′ cirrhosis	Miyake's type A′ cirrhosis
Macroscopic characteristics of completed stage	Broad stromal, micro- to macronodular atrophic cirrhosis	Thin stromal, macro-nodular atrophic cirrhosis	Thin stromal, macro-nodular atrophic cir-rhosis
Incidence in Japan[b]	ca. 5%	ca. 75%	ca. 10%
Association of hepatocellular carcinoma	Scarce	Frequent	Low

[a]International synonyms are indicated in parenthesis; [b]At the present time the common type of cirrhosis comprises about 90% of all the cirrhosis in Japan, whilst the specific type of cirrhosis is less than 10% in incidence.

thin stromal connective tissue stroma are characteristic findings (Fig. 8). Multi-lobular pseudolobule formation with scanty hepatocellular damage, few inflammatory cells infiltrated into connective tissue stroma, and newly formed thick elastic fibers encircling the pseudolobules are histopathological hallmarks (Fig. 9). The high-association incidence of hepatocellular carcinoma is also a hallmark of type B cirrhosis (*cf.* Table 2).

Miyake's type F cirrhosis is compatible with alcoholic cirrhosis, and has been called fatty and/or nutritional cirrhosis. In a typical case, the liver is hypertrophic and regularly micronodular pseudolobule formation with thin connective tissue stroma is a characteristic finding (Fig. 10). In cases in an advanced stage, the liver becomes atrophic and associated with postnecrotic features. Histologically, hepatocytes in and around the pseudolobules are usually severely infiltrated with large fat droplets (Fig. 11). Alcoholic hyalin can be detected in hepatocytes, however, hyalin bodies are not so common in Japanese cases. Connective tissue stroma contain a small number of inflammatory cells and few thin elastic fibers. In

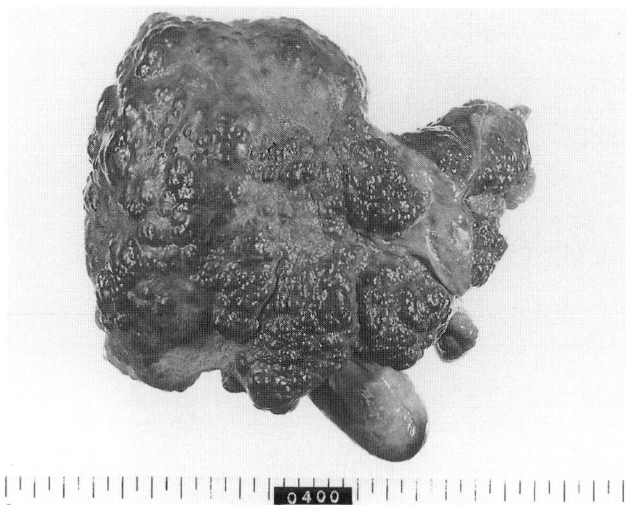

Fig. 5. Nagayo-Miyake's type A liver cirrhosis. Extensive areas of collapse are recognizable and pseudolobules are irregular in size. This type of cirrhosis is compatible with postnecrotic cirrhosis.

spite of a decrease in the amount of hepatic parenchyma in alcoholic cirrhosis, most cases of alcoholic cirrhosis are macroscopically hypertrophic due to abundant fat infiltration of hepatocytes. This condition is very similar to the pseudo-

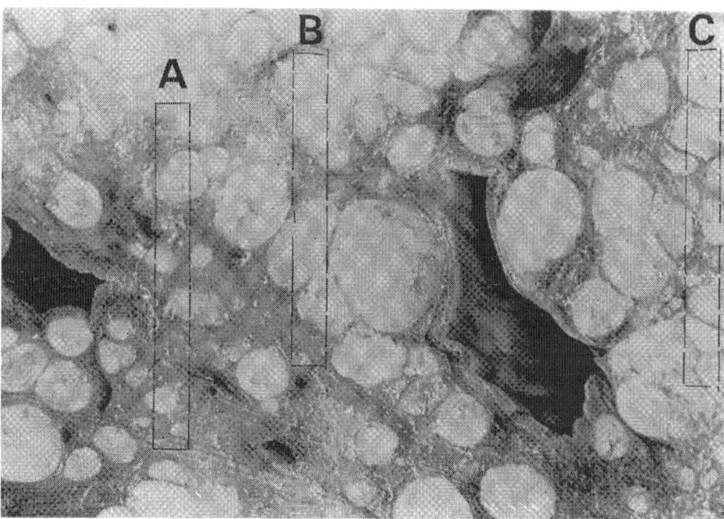

Fig. 6. A Macroscopical finding of a cut surface of Nagayo-Miyake's type A cirrhosis. Pseudolobules are irregular in size, and connective tissue stroma is broad. Markedly distorted large hepatic veins are recognizable. When needle biopsy materials are taken from three different portions (indicated with cylinders A, B and C) for histopathologic examinations, the histologic diagnosis may be different from each other.

8

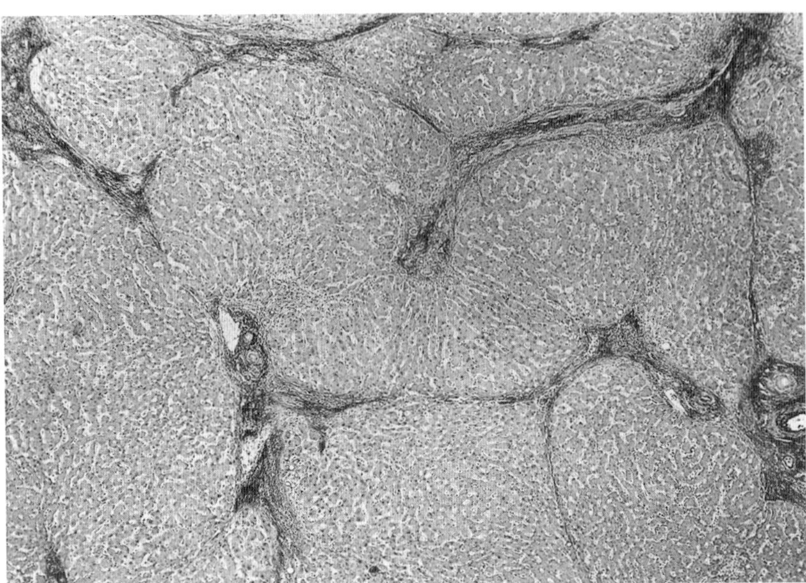

Fig. 7. A Histological finding of Miyake's type B' cirrhosis. This type is in the precirrhotic stage of Nagayo-Miyake's type B cirrhosis and is compatible with incomplete septal cirrhosis. There is fibrotic septa linking with neighboring portal tracts and occasionally with central veins. However, pseudo-lobular disorganization is not completed. Elastica van Gieson stain, X32.

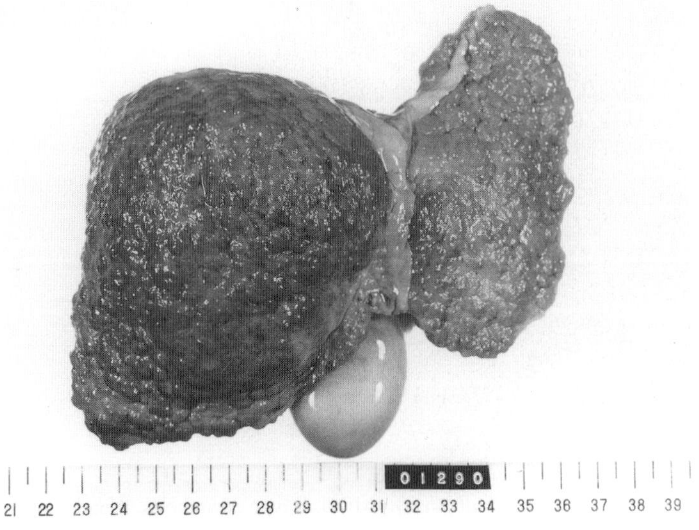

Fig. 8. Nagayo-Miyake's type B liver cirrhosis. Macroscopically, the liver is atrophic, and a majority of pseudolobules are 5–6 mm in diameter. This type is almost identical to posthepatitic cirrhosis and macronodular cirrhosis.

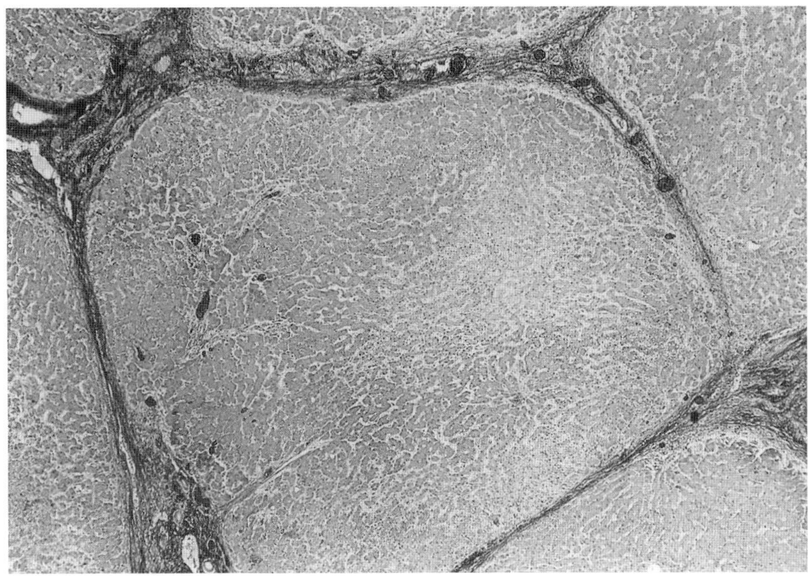

Fig. 9. A histological finding of Nagayo-Miyake's type B cirrhosis. Multilobular, large pseudolobules are surrounded by thin stromal connective tissue. The borderline of the pseudolobules is sharp and distinct.

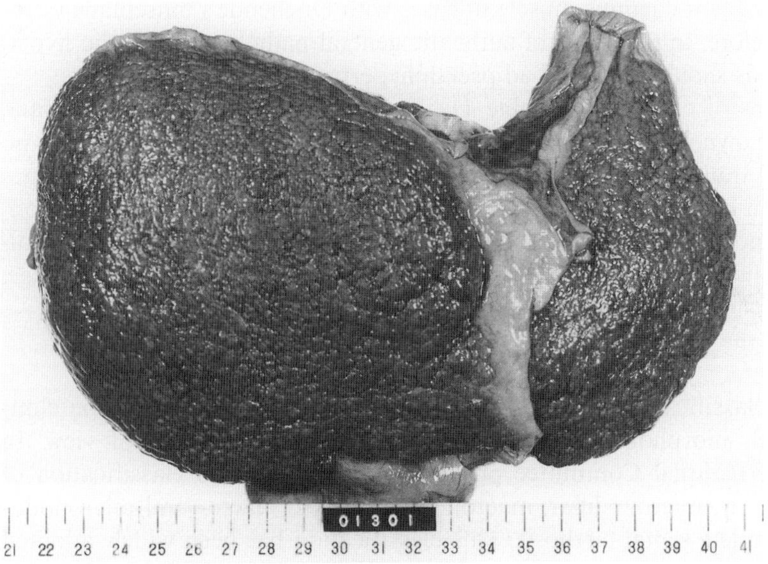

Fig. 10. The naked eye appearance of Miyake's type F cirrhosis. The liver is rather hypertrophic and the micronodular pseudolobules are less than three mm in size. This type of cirrhosis is compatible with alcoholic cirrhosis.

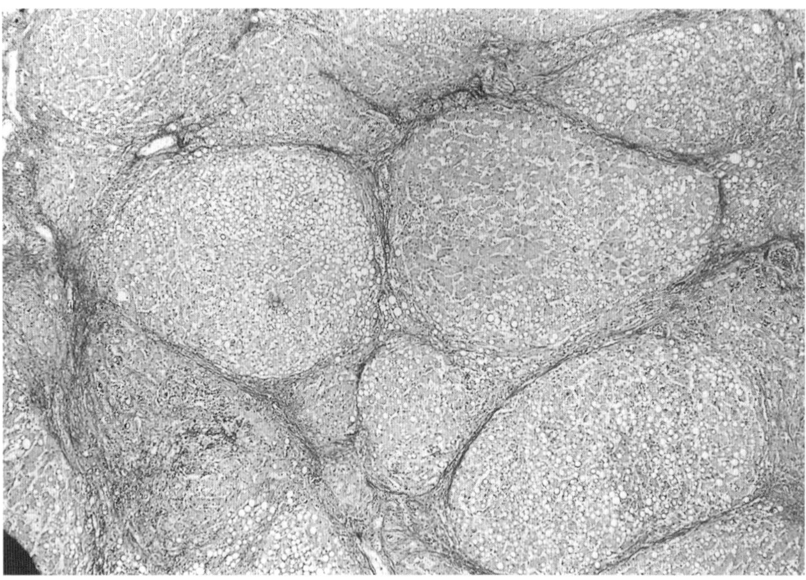

Fig. 11. A histopathological view of Miyake's type F cirrhosis. Micronodular, mostly sublobular pseudolobules are surrounded by thin stromal connective tissue, in which the elastic fibers (seen as fine and black lines in this figure) are scanty. Hepatic parenchymal cells indicate marked fatty change. Elastica van Gieson stain, X32.

hypertrophy of gastrocnemius muscle in cases with Duchenne's muscular dystrophy [12]. Therefore, in the sense of authentic general pathology, alcoholic hypertrophic cirrhosis should be called ad pseudohypertrophic cirrhosis.

Specific types of cirrhosis (*cf.* Table 1), i.e., congestive, biliary, and parasitia, etc., have their own etiology and peculiar morphogenesis, respectively, and so no morphological transition is detectable amongst them. Diagnosis of specific types of cirrhosis can be made even in the early stage of the cirrhotic process. In contrast, the diagnosis of the common type of cirrhosis is only applicable to a completed and/or fully developed stage of cirrhosis, and not to the precirrhotic stage.

Comments on the classification of cirrhosis

A number of classifications of liver cirrhosis have been proposed from the clinical, etiological, morphogenetical, and morbid anatomical points of view. In 1979, the International Committee proposed a morphological classification of liver cirrhosis, i.e., micronodular, macronodular, mixed macro- and micronodular, and incomplete septal cirrhosis. This classification has been widely adopted throughout the world.

It has been widely recognized that the size of pseudonodules and the width of connective tissue stroma are not uniform in a given case of liver cirrhosis. This is true of most cases of liver cirrhosis. Therefore, morphologic classification of liver cirrhosis should principally be based upon the predominant type of both the size of pseudonodules and the width of connective tissue stroma. Thus, it is reasonable to assume that autopsy diagnosis based upon macroscopical scrutiny of entire liver and/or peritoneoscopic diagnosis could be more accurate and better than needle biopsy diagnosis.

Clinical signs and symptoms in patients with liver cirrhosis could be explained by the following three principal morphological changes: volumetric decrease in hepatocytes, parenchymal, stromal and vascular architectural alterations, and decrease in sinusoidal blood flow.

Is liver cirrhosis incurable? Before trying to answer this question, I would like to point out a peculiar finding concerning the connective tissue stroma of liver cirrhosis. In contrast to the hyalinized scar tissue in old myocardial infarctions and in a base of chronic gastric ulcers, no hyalinized scar tissue could be detected in most of the connective tissue stroma of liver cirrhosis, even in advanced cases. Moreover, as in experimental liver cirrhosis, when the administration of an etiologic agent is stopped and normal diet is given continuously, the cirrhotic change will reverse and change into a normal liver. From this evidence, it is conceivable that liver cirrhosis is not an irreversible and/or incurable disease, I would like to stress that liver cirrhosis might principally be a curable condition of the liver.

For the successive treatment of liver cirrhosis, stopping the continuous and repetitious necrosis of hepatocytes, and a quantitative and qualitative increase of sinusoidal blood flow will be essential.

Conclusion

The classification of liver cirrhosis in Japan is presented. Nagayo-Miyake's classification of the common types of liver cirrhosis is popular in Japan, and its morbid anatomical findings are demonstrated briefly.

It is my hope that liver cirrhosis is not assumed to be an end stage and/or noncurable condition of the liver, and will become a curable hepatic disease in the coming 21st century.

Reference

1. Galambos JT. Cirrhosis. Philadelphia: W.B. Saunders, 1979.
2. Laennec RTH. De l'auscultation médiate 2nd edn. Paris: Brosson et Chaude, 1826;2:196.
3. Nagayo M. Liver cirrhosis. Morbid anatomical study (in Japanese). Tr Soc Pathol Jpn 1914;4: 31—72.
4. Japanese Pathological Society (eds) Annual of Pathological Autopsy Cases in Japan, 1992, vol 35.
5. Okudaira M. Liver Pathology for Clinic (in Japanese). Japan: Igaku Shoin, 1995.
6. Miyake M, Amano S, Kosaka S et al. Morphologic criteria of liver cirrhosis (in Japanese). Acta Hepatol Jpn 1965;6:177—182.
7. Okudaira M. Anatomy of the portal vein system and hepatic vasculature. In: Okuda K, Benhamou JP (eds) Hypertension. Tokyo: Springer-Verlag, 1991;3—12.
8. Miyake M, Saito M, Okudaira M. Studies on hepatic vascular alteration in cirrhosis of the liver. Jpn Cir J 1964;28:33—39.

9. Miyake M. Pathology of the liver, especially on cirrhosis (in Japanese). Tr Soc Pathol Jpn 1960; 49:589−632.
10. Mori W. Classification of liver cirrhosis (in Japanese). Igaku No Ayumi 1964;48:371−381.
11. Leavy CM, Popper H, Sherlock S. Diseases of the Liver and Biliary Tract. Standardization of Nomenclature, Diagnostic Criteria, and Diagnostic Methodology. London: Castle House Publ., 1979.
12. Daniel PM, Strich SJ, Harriman DGF. Skeletal Muscle. In: Symmers W St C et al. (eds) Systemic Pathology, vol 5, 2nd edn. Edinburgh: Churchill, 1979;2358−2359.

Etiology of liver cirrhosis in an urban population in Japan

Hisato Nakajima, Ichiro Takagi, Masayoshi Yamauchi and Gotaro Toda

Department of Internal Medicine 1, The Jikei University School of Medicine, Minato-ku, Tokyo, Japan

Abstract. To clarify the etiology of liver cirrhosis in Japan, we analyzed 779 patients with liver cirrhosis in Jikei University School of Medicine in Tokyo. Etiology was Hepatitis C virus (HCV), 58.8%; Hepatitis B virus (HBV), 10.9%; HBV+HCV, 2.8%; alcohol, 9.4%; HCV+alcohol, 5.5%; non-B non-C (NBNC), 5.4%; and primary biliary cirrhosis (PBC), 7.4% in the Tokyo area. The top three causes in male patients were HCV at 57.6%, HBV at 13.8%, and alcohol at 12.3%, while those in females were HCV at 61.9%, PBC at 17.4%, and NBNC at 9.6%. Furthermore, the top three causes in patients under 59 years of age were HCV at 43.5%, HBV at 17.7%, and alcohol at 15%. In patients over 60 years of age, HCV was more than 72%. Compared with other areas of Japan, the incidence of HCV in Tokyo was higher, while that of HBV and alcohol were lower. This distribution was similar to that in the Tohoku region of northern Japan. Using multilogistic model analysis, HCV was found to be the highest risk factor for hepatocellular carcinoma in patients with liver cirrhosis. Thus, the most common etiology of liver cirrhosis and major risk factor of hepatocellular carcinoma was HCV.

Keywords: cirrhosis, hepatitis B virus, hepatitis C virus, hepatocellular carcinoma.

Introduction

In Asia, the carrier rate of hepatitis B virus (HBV) is 3—5%, and 6—10% in Southeast Asia [1]. In Southeast Asia, the carrier rate of hepatitis C virus (HCV) is also high, at 4—8% [2—5]. In Japan, the carrier rate of HBV and HCV are about 1—2% [1,6]. These rates are higher than those in Europe and North America, where HBV is under 0.1% [1], and HCV is under 1% [5]. Furthermore, annual alcohol (100% ethanol) consumption in Europe is about 10—13 l per person, about 1.5 times higher than that in Japan [7].

These facts suggest that the etiology of chronic liver disease in Japan, largely due to hepatitis virus, is quite different from that in North America and Europe. In this study, we investigated the etiology of liver cirrhosis in patients who visited Jikei University Hospital.

Materials and Methods

A total of 779 patients with liver cirrhosis treated at Jikei University School Hospital between 1990 and 1996 were analyzed (Table 1).

Address for correspondence: Hisato Nakajima MD, Department of Internal Medicine 1, Jikei University School of Medicine, 25-8, 3-Chome, Nishi-Shinbashi, Minato-ku, Tokyo 105-8461, Japan.

14

Table 1. Background of patients with liver cirrhosis.

	Number of patients	Age of patients (years)
Male	556	59 ± 9.7
Female	223	62 ± 9.8

Liver cirrhosis was diagnosed by a combination of laparoscopy, ultrasound, radioisotope scanning, CT scan and biopsy.

The etiology of cirrhosis was divided into eight groups, namely hepatitis B virus (HBV), hepatitis C virus (HCV), HBV+HCV, alcohol, HBV+alcohol, HCV+alcohol, non-B non-C (NBNC) and primary biliary cirrhosis (PBC). "HBV" means positive HBs antigen, "HCV" means positive anti-HCV antibody or HCV-RNA, "HBV+HCV" means double infection with HBV and HCV, "alcohol" means daily ethanol intake over 24 g during the last 10 years, "HBV+alcohol" means HBV infection and alcoholic liver damage, "HCV+alcohol" means HCV infection and alcoholic liver damage, "NBNC" means negative reaction for HBs antigen and anti-HCV antibody or HCV-RNA, and "PBC" means only stage IV disease.

Etiology of liver cirrhosis was analyzed according to total patient number and divided into sex and age groups. Annual changes in etiology year by year between 1990 and 1996 were also analyzed. Furthermore, risk factors for hepatocellular carcinoma (HCC) were investigated using the multilogistic model.

Results

Etiology of liver cirrhosis in the Jikei University School of Medicine

The Jikei University is located in the middle of Tokyo City, and treats 981 patients with chronic hepatitis (CH), 419 patients with liver cirrhosis (LC), 307 patients with fatty liver (FL) and 299 patients with chronic liver disease and HCC monthly.

As shown in Fig. 1, etiology in 779 patients with liver cirrhosis was HCV in 58.8%, HBV 10.9%, HBV+HCV 2.8%, alcohol 9.4%, HCV+alcohol 5.5%, non-B non-C, 5.4%, and PBC 7.4%. The mean age was 51.3 years for male and 59.4 years for female HBV sufferers, 61.7 years for male and 63.6 years for female HCV sufferers, and 56.0 years for male and 57.2 years for female PBC sufferers.

Distribution of etiology by sex

Etiology in males was HCV in 57.6%, HBV 13.8%, alcohol 12.3%, HCV+alcohol 6.8%, NBNC 3.7%, HBV+HCV 2.9%, and PBC, while that in females was HCV 61.9%, PBC 17.4%, non-B non-C 9.6%, HBV 3.7%, alcohol 2.3%, HCV+alcohol 2.3%, and HBV+HCV 2.3% (Fig. 2). In females, the incidence of

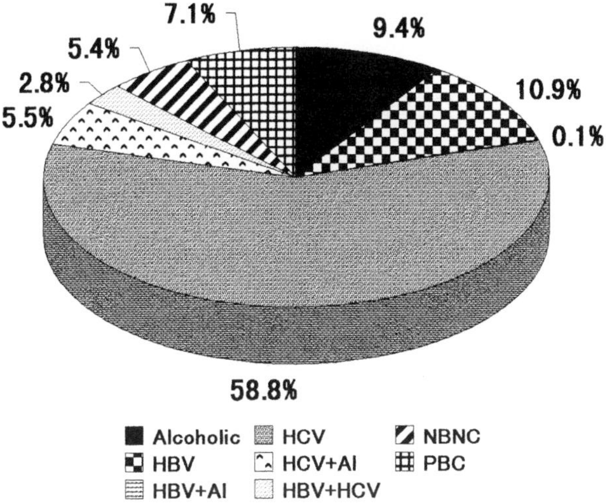

Fig. 1. Etiology of cirrhosis in the Jikei University School of Medicine.

HCV, PBC and NBNC was higher, and alcohol, HBV and HCV+alcohol were lower than that in males.

Distribution of etiology by age

Etiology in patients under 59 years of age was HCV in 43.5%, HBV 17.7%, alcohol 15%, PBC 9.3%, HCV+alcohol 6.9%, NBNC 4.5%, and HBV+HCV 2.7%. However, in patients aged 60 years or older, etiology was HCV in 72.0%, NBNC 6.0%, alcohol 5.0%, HBV 5.0%, PBC 5.0%, HCV+alcohol 4.3%, and

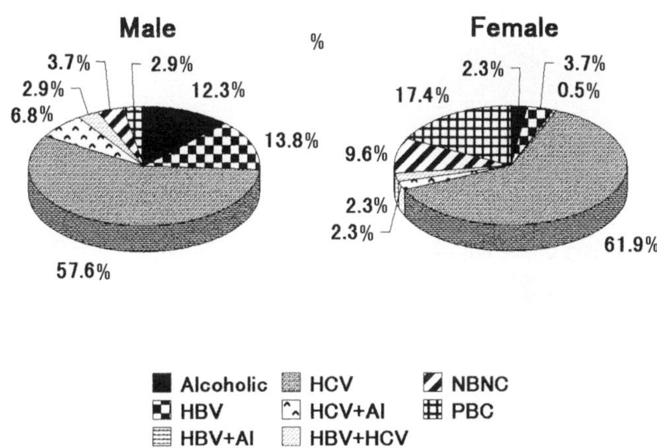

Fig. 2. Etiology of cirrhosis classified by sex.

16

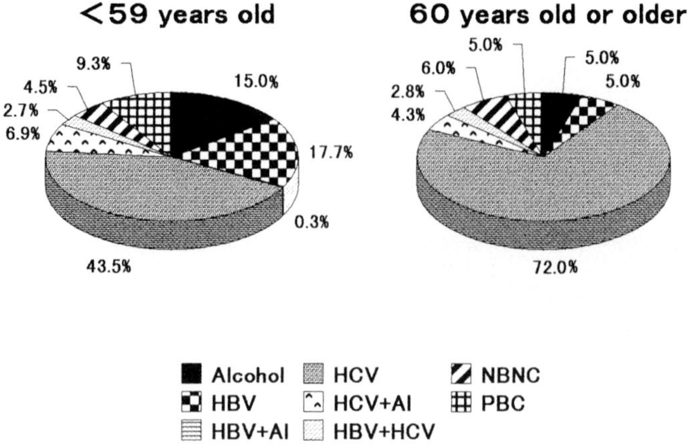

Fig. 3. Etiology of cirrhosis classified according to age.

HBV+HCV 2.8% (Fig. 3). Compared with the under-59 age group, HCV in the over-60 years age group was 1.5 times higher, though HBV, alcohol and PBC were lower. As shown in Fig. 4, incidence of HCV was greatest in all age and sex groups. Rate of HCV was highest in females over 60 years, and second in males over 60 years. Rate of alcohol was highest in males under 59 years and second in males over 60 years. The rate of HBV was highest in males under 59 years of age, that of PBC was highest in females under 59 years of age, and that of NBNC was highest in females over 60 years of age.

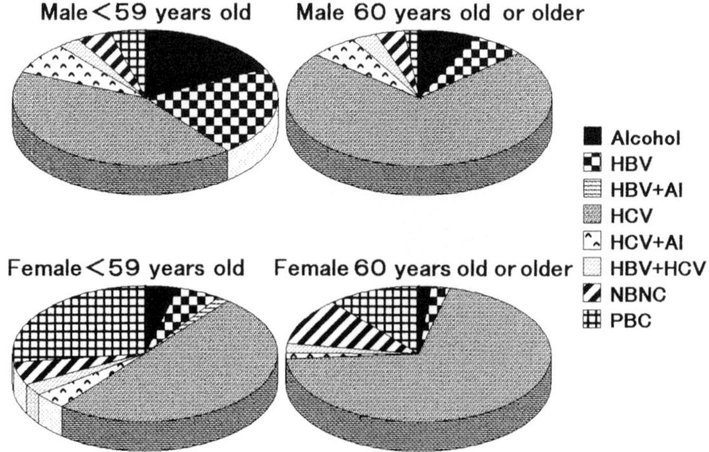

Fig. 4. Etiology of cirrhosis classified by sex and age.

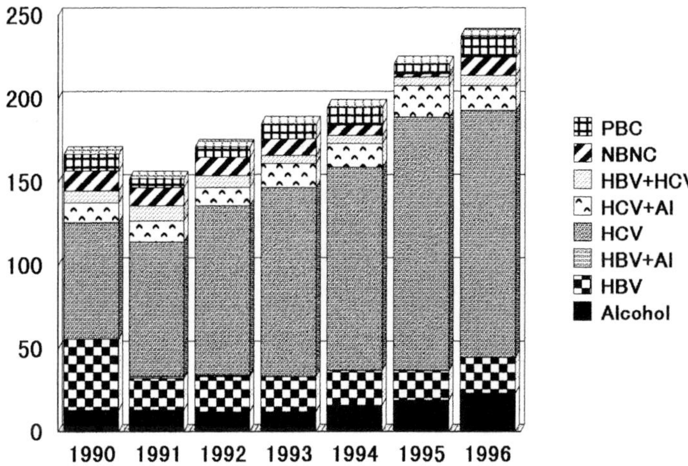

Fig. 5. Annual changes in distribution of etiology in patients with cirrhosis.

Annual change in distribution of etiology

From 1990 to 1996, the number of patients with cirrhosis increased each year, especially that due to HCV (Fig. 5). Alcohol-induced cirrhosis increased slightly, and that due to HBV tended to decrease. Figure 6 shows annual changes in the rate of each etiology. These percentages reflect changes in the number of patients

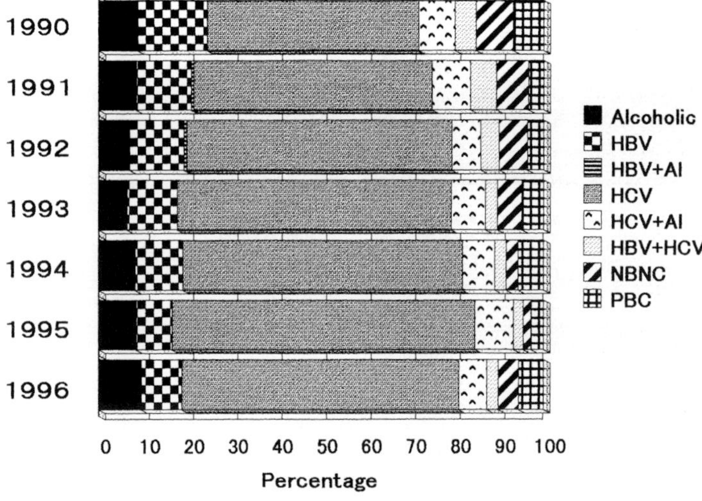

Fig. 6. Annual changes in distribution of etiology in cirrhosis.

18

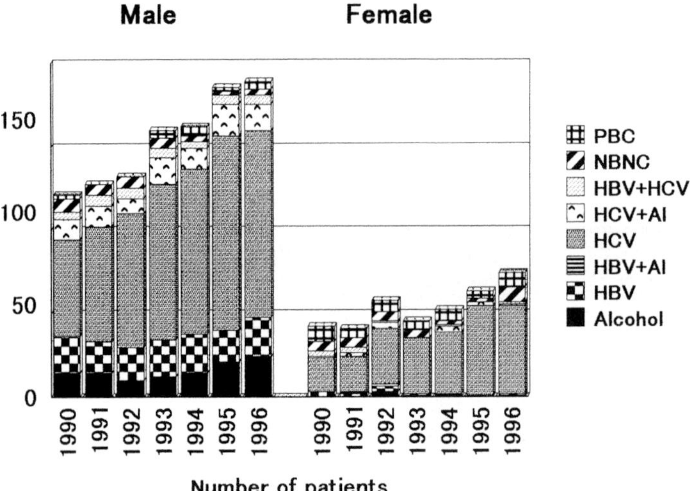

Fig. 7. Annual change in distribution of etiology in patients with cirrhosis classified by sex.

(Fig. 5). The rate of HCV became very high. Figures 7 and 8 show the annual change in the number and percentage of each etiology classified by sex. HCV was the major factor in both males and females. In males, HCV and alcohol increased, while HBV and NBNC decreased. In females, HCV in particular increased and HBV, HBV+HCV and NBNC decreased.

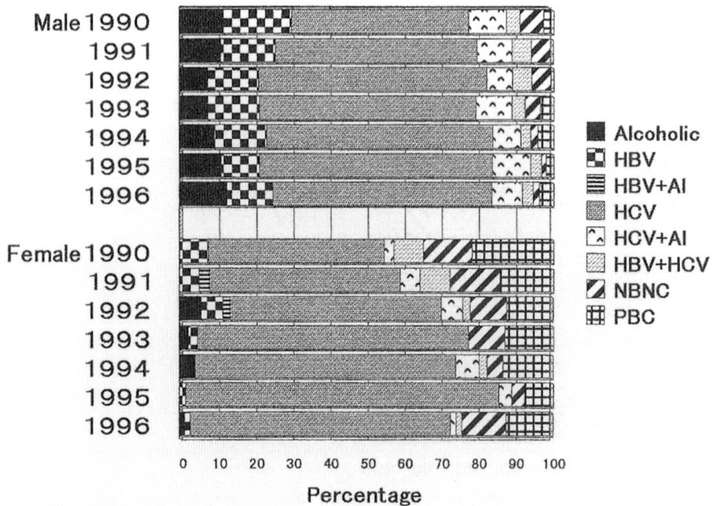

Fig. 8. Annual change in distribution of etiology in cirrhosis classified by sex.

Risk factors for HCC

In 779 patients with cirrhosis, 351 of 556 males and 95 of 223 females had HCC. The mean age for type B HCC was for males 54.3 years and females 63.8 years ($p < 0.005$), type C HCC 63.2 years and 65.0 years ($p < 0.025$), HCV+alcohol 61.2 years and 56 years, HBV+HCV 58.5 years and 68 years, NBNC 62.4 and 71.7 years ($p < 0.05$), respectively. The risk factors of HCC in these patients were identified using a multilogistic model. As shown in Table 2, the greatest factor was HCV ($p < 0.0000$), followed by HBV ($p < 0.0000$), NBNC ($p < 0.0013$) and HBV+HCV ($p < 0.0027$) in descending rank. HBV+alcohol and HCV+alcohol could not be calculated because of the small number of patients. Alcohol was not recognized as a risk factor for HCC. There was no correlation between alcohol and HCC.

Discussion

Cirrhosis is a serious and irreversible disease and the end result of chronic hepatocellular injury. In district general hospitals in the UK, 80% of all cases of cirrhosis are associated with alcohol [8]. In the USA, cirrhosis is the 11th leading cause of death, with an age-adjusted death rate of 9.2 per 100,000 per year with over 45% of cases being alcohol-related [9]. Deaths from cirrhosis, mostly alcohol-related, increased by 72% between 1950 and 1974, making it the fourth most common cause of death in white male adults [8]. The present study suggests that the etiology of cirrhosis in Europe and the USA is very different from that of Japan. In Japan, incidence due to alcohol was about 10—20%, while 75—85% was due to hepatitis virus. In Europe and the USA, 50—80% was due to alcohol, a rate much higher than that in Japan.

Because this study was conducted in a single institution, etiology rates may not reflect average etiology in Japan. Jikei University is located in central Tokyo, and over 70% of patients are white-collar businessmen and their families. From this study, etiology due to alcohol was 9.4%, hence the alcohol intake of these businessmen was not high, and alcohol was a low-grade risk factor for cirrhosis.

Incidence of cirrhosis due to alcohol, HBV, NBNC and PBC was sex-related, while that due to HCV, HBV, alcohol and PBC was age-related. HCV increased annually while HBV decreased. Thus, incidence due to HBV decreased relatively

Table 2. Risk factors for HCC analyzed using a multilogistic model.

Variable name	Coefficient	Standard error	t value	F value	p value
HBV	1.743702	0.332079	5.251	27.572	0.00001
HCV	1.850372	0.261859	7.066	49.932	0.00001
Alcohol	−0.852996	0.446557	−1.911	3.649	0.05649
HBV+HCV	1.514128	0.503222	3.009	9.053	0.00271
Non-B non-C	1.275236	0.395483	3.225	10.397	0.00132

20

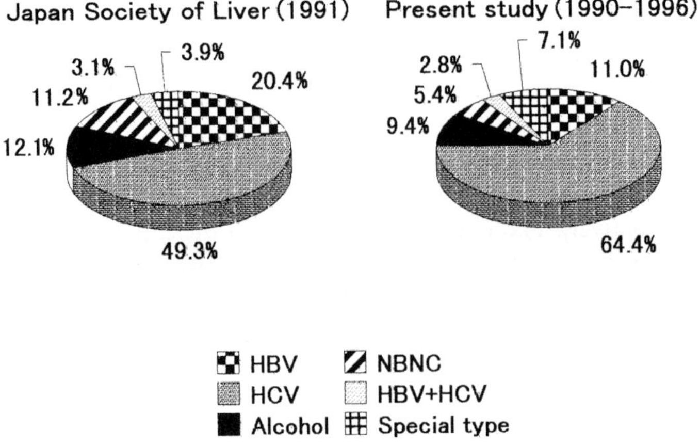

Fig. 9. Comparison of etiology of cirrhosis with a previous study.

to that by HCV. The rate of NBNC might be a course of development of diagnostic methods.

Figures 9 and 10 compare this study (1990–1996) with a report by the Japanese Society of Liver in 1991 [10]. In this study, the increase of HCV and decrease of HBV, alcohol and NBNC were characteristic. Figure 10 shows the results of etiology in eight regions and in this study. Percentage of HCV was the highest, HBV, NBNC and alcohol were lower than that of another region. This distribution was similar to that in the Tohoku region of northern Japan.

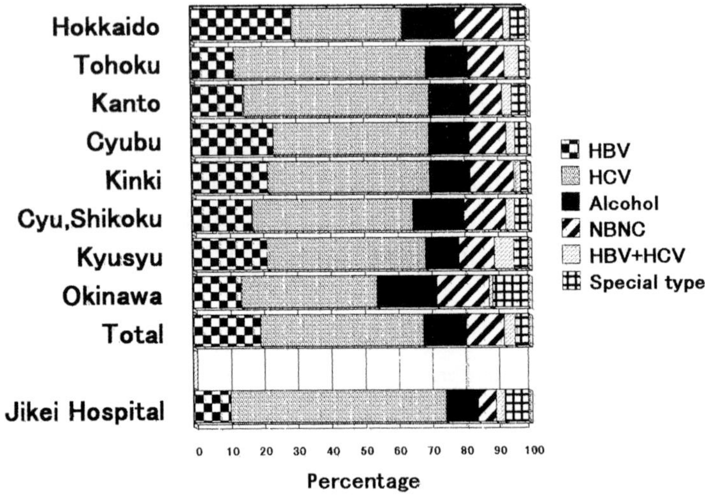

Fig. 10. Etiology of cirrhosis in Japan by region. Compared with Japan Society of Liver Study (1991).

Using a multilogistic model analysis, HCV was the highest risk factor for hepatocellular carcinoma in patients with liver cirrhosis.

Thus, HCV was the major etiology of liver cirrhosis and the greatest risk factor for hepatocellular carcinoma in Tokyo, Japan.

References

1. Sobeslavsky O. Prevalence of markers of hepatitis B virus infection in various countries: a WHO collaborative study. Bull World Health Organ 1980;58:621–628.
2. Contreras M, Barbara JA, Anderson C, Ranasinghe E, Moore C, Brennan MT et al. Low incidence of non-A, non-B post-transfusion hepatitis in London confirmed by hepatitis C virus serology. Lancet 1991;337:357–364.
3. Williams AE, Dodd RY. The serology of hepatitis C virus in relation to post-transfusion hepatitis. Ann Clin Lab Sci 1990;20:192–199.
4. Esteban JI, Gonzales A, Hernandez JE, Viladomiu L, Sanches C, Talavera JCL et al. Evaluation of antibody to hepatitis C virus. A study of transfusion-associated hepatitis. N Engl J Med 1990;323:1107–1112.
5. Sirchia G, Almini D, Bellobuono A. Prevalence of hepatitis C virus antibodies in Italian blood donors. Vox Sang 1990;59:26–29.
6. Tanaka E, Kiyosawa K, Sodeyama T, Hayata T, Ohike Y, Nakano Y et al. Prevalence of antibody to hepatitis C virus in Japanese school children: comparison with adult blood donors. Am J Trop Med Hyg 1992;46:460–464.
7. Harada T. Etiology of cirrhosis. J Jpn Soc Int Med 1991;80:1563–1567.
8. Eddleston ALWF. Chronic alcoholic liver disease. In: Souhami RL, Moxham J (eds) Textbook of Medicine. New York: Churchill Livingstone, 1990;644–645.
9. Friedman LS. Cirrhosis. In: Tierney LM, McPhee SJ, Papadakis MA (eds) Current Medical Diagnosis and Treatment. Stamford: A Simon & Schuster Company, 1997;620–621.
10. Harada T, Kobayashi K. Discussion about etiology of liver cirrhosis. In: Ora Y, Harada T, Kobayashi K (eds) Etiologies of Liver Cirrhosis in Japanese Population. Tokyo: Nihon Igakukun, 1991;175–193.

1998 Elsevier Science B.V.
Progress in Hepatology, Volume 4.
Liver Cirrhosis Update.
M. Yamanaka et al., editors.

Molecular pathology of liver fibrosis

Isao Okazaki[1], Tetsu Watanabe[1], Shigenari Hozawa[1] and Katsuya Maruyama[2]
*[1]Department of Community Health, School of Medicine, Tokai University, Isehara, Kanagawa; and
[2]Department of Medicine, Kurihama National Hospital, Kanagawa, Japan*

Abstract. Recent advances in the understanding of molecular pathophysiology of hepatic fibrosis, especially (1) the mechanism of activation of Ito cells, (2) the analysis of promoter regions of extracellular matrix biosynthesis, and (3) the role of matrix metalloproteinases (MMPs) and their specific inhibitors (TIMPs, tissue inhibitors of MMPs) in the formation of and the recovery from liver fibrosis were reviewed. It has been known that Ito cells are activated via the expression of c-myb and NFκB which is induced by oxidative stress, and inhibited by antioxidant (1-α-tocopherol) and butylated hydroxytoluene. The activation mechanism is now being revealed. TGF-β stimulates the human COL1A2 (α2 chain of type I collagen) gene transcription by increasing the affinity of an Sp1-containing transcriptional complex bound to an upstream sequence termed the TGF-β-responsive element. Inagaki et al. obtained two passage-possible clones of CFSC-2G, and CFSC-5H from primary cultures of rat Ito cells in fibrotic livers, and developed a transgenic mouse which made it possible to monitor the promoter activity of COL1A2 gene in the process of hepatic fibrogenesis. It has been also clarified that activated Ito cells can produce matrix components as well as MMPs. Very recently the authors observed the participation of MMP-1 (matrix metalloproteinase-1) in the recovery from experimental hepatic fibrosis using RT-PCR and in situ hybridization. MMPs should be investigated in order to clarify the mechanism of matrix degradation seen in the recovery from liver fibrosis experimentally and clinically.

Keywords: activation of Ito cells, Ito cells, matrix metalloproteinases (MMPs), myofibroblast, promoter gene of COL1A2 (α2 chain of type I collagen), tissue inhibitor of MMPs (TIMPs).

Introduction

During the past 10 years we have had several excellent reviews on hepatic fibrogenesis of which molecular mechanisms have been extensively studied [1–6]. However, the description of collagen degradation in the liver is still limited [4–6]. The reversibility of liver fibrosis has been observed clinically by physicians. Rubin and Hutterer [7] reported on cases which recovered from alcoholic liver fibrosis by abstinence. Perez-Tamayo described an interesting case of hemochromatosis, where surgical biopsy showed liver cirrhosis. After ^{32}P treatment, the patient recovered from hemochromatosis, and a second biopsy revealed a pathologically normal liver [8]. There were, however, very few cases showing recovery from hepatic fibrosis as evidenced by morphological observation [9]. Cameron and Karunaratne pathologically demonstrated the reversibility of liver fibrosis of rats experimentally induced by chronic carbon tetrachloride intoxication [10].

Address for correspondence: Isao Okazaki MD, PhD, Department of Community Health, Tokai University School of Medicine, Isehara, Kanagawa 259-1193, Japan.

24

On the basis of the finding of "Collagenase activity in experimental hepatic fibrosis" [11] the authors and their colleagues have been studying the role of collagenase expression and metabolisms on molecular mechanisms of reversibility of liver fibrosis [12—23] in the hope of solving the question "How can we treat and recover from liver cirrhosis?"

The research on liver fibrosis has advanced with molecular biological techniques for the past few years. In this review, the authors focus on the three following recent advances, including their recent findings from the view points of molecular biology and pathology:
1) the mechanism of Ito cells activation,
2) the characterization of promoter region of COL1A2 in Ito cells, and
3) the role of MMPs in recovery from liver fibrosis.

Mechanism of Ito cells activation

Ito cells (hepatic stellate cells, fat-storing cells, lipocytes) have been reported to be responsible for extracellular matrix production under pathological conditions [2]. Takahara et al. [24] observed that Ito cells are positive for monoclonal antibodies against several types of collagens and several other extracellular matrix components. Subsequent in situ hybridization studies by Milani et al. [25] revealed that mRNAs for COL1A2, $\alpha 1$ chain of type III collagen, and $\alpha 1$ chain of type IV collagen are expressed at the mesenchymal cells in the portal tracts and at the perisinusoidal cells and the mesenchymal cells around the periphery of veins and arteries, but not in hepatocytes. Biochemical studies further confirmed that Ito cells are responsible for the major production of extracellular matrix [26]. For example, Armendariz-Borunda et al. observed TGF-β gene expression in both parenchymal and nonparenchymal cells after chronic carbon tetrachloride treatment and found increased expression of TGF-β gene expression in nonparenchymal cells after 2 to 3 weeks of treatment [26].

In vitro studies using cultured Ito cells by electron microscopy [1—3] revealed that Ito cells transformed to myofibroblasts that could be potential cells for extracellular matrix production. This transformation is known as an activation of Ito cells. Figure 1 shows the potential triggers for activation of Ito cells and phenotypic changes occurred with activation. This review focuses on the molecular and pathological changes of activated Ito cells.

Ito cells are activated via the expression of c-myb and NFκB which is induced by oxidative stress. There is evidence from the following observations. Lee et al. [27] demonstrated that Ito cells were activated by the generation of free radicals by ascorbate/FeSO$_4$ and by malondialdehyde, a product of lipid peroxidation. Ito cells were also activated by type I collagen and TGF-α. This activation was inhibited by antioxidant (1-α-tocopherol) and butylated hydroxytoluene. These valuable findings are explained by the fact that oxidative stress, TGF-α, and collagen type I caused proliferation of activated Ito cells by NFκB and c-myb. Antioxidant and c-myb antisense oligonucleotide inhibited both type I collagen and

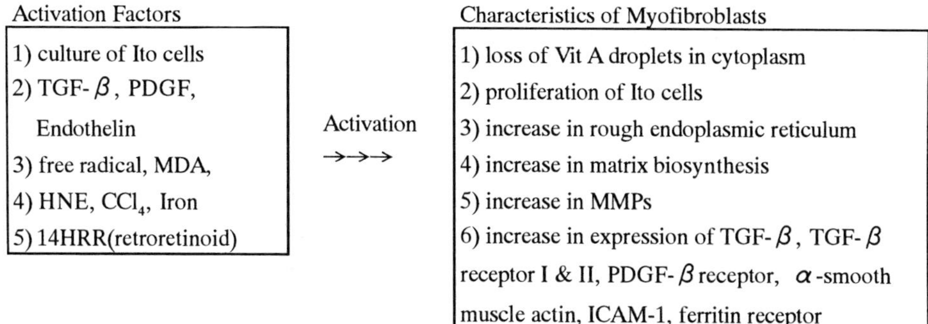

Activation Factors		Characteristics of Myofibroblasts
1) culture of Ito cells		1) loss of Vit A droplets in cytoplasm
2) TGF-β, PDGF,		2) proliferation of Ito cells
Endothelin	Activation	3) increase in rough endoplasmic reticulum
3) free radical, MDA,	$\rightarrow\rightarrow\rightarrow$	4) increase in matrix biosynthesis
4) HNE, CCl$_4$, Iron		5) increase in MMPs
5) 14HRR(retroretinoid)		6) increase in expression of TGF-β, TGF-β receptor I & II, PDGF-β receptor, α-smooth muscle actin, ICAM-1, ferritin receptor

Fig. 1. Activation factors of Ito cells and characteristics which appeared of myofibroblasts.

TGF-α-induced activation of Ito cells. Moreover, these materials inhibited not only the expression of NFκB and c-myb, but also the proliferation of activated Ito cells (myofibroblasts) [27]. Lee et al. further demonstrated that promoter E box of α-smooth muscle actin gene extracted from nuclear fraction of the activated Ito cells was disrupted by antibodies to NFκB65 and c-myb. c-myb was also expressed in the activated Ito cells of fibrotic liver in rats induced by the chronic administration of carbon tetrachloride [27].

Another series of interesting reports derives from the research of nuclear transcription activity of retinoid X receptor (RXR) and/or retinoic acid receptor (RAR) α, β, γ in reaction with retinoic acid. Weiner et al. [28] revealed that RARβ mRNA expression was observed at Ito cells isolated from normal rat liver, but not observed at the activated Ito cells from fibrotic liver, although cellular retinol-binding protein (CRBP) mRNA expression was increased in the activated Ito cells. Decreased expression of RARβ mRNA in the activated Ito cells was recovered by the administration of retinoic acid or retinoyl acetate [28].

Very recently Okuno et al. found that 9, 13-di-cis-retinoic acid activates Ito cells [29]. They observed that this new retinoic acid bound RAR receptor and increased gene expression of plasminogen activator, TGF-β2 and TGF-β3, as well as type I procollagen. They postulated that the activation of plasmin activity on cell surface may regulate the activation of latent TGF-β which, in turn, causes liver fibrosis [29].

Endothelin induced the activation of Ito cells, and antagonist of endothelin (bosentan) inhibited the activation of Ito cells [30]. PDGF has been known as a cytokine to stimulate collagen production, and pentoxifylline is now noted as a inhibitor of PDGF and also as an inhibitor of the activation of Ito cells [31]. A recent paper by Marra et al. [32] clarified the participation of phosphatidylinositol 3-kinase in the pathway of the activation of Ito cells by PDGF, and revealed that this phosphorylation is necessary for the motility, proliferation and transformation of Ito cells to myofibroblasts.

Characterization of promoter region of COL1A2 gene

Inagaki et al. identified the promoter region of COL1A2 gene and reported that TGF-β stimulates the human COL1A2 gene by increasing the affinity of an Sp1-containing transcriptional complex bound to an upstream sequence termed the TGF-β-responsive element [33]. The TGF-β-responsive element in the COL1A2 promoter located at 131 bp upstream has at least two cis-acting elements. TGF-β-responsive element contained neighboring protein-bound sequences, termed Box 3A and Box B. They found that an Sp1 recognition sequence existed within Box 3A, and that a functional interaction between Sp1 and other components of the TGF-β-responsive element complex may mediate the stimulation of COL1A2 gene expression by TGFβ. Moreover, they reported that the TGF-β-responsive element-bound complex mediates the inhibitory signal of TNF-α [34].

They established two passage-possible clones of CFSC-2G and CFSC-5H from primary cultures of Ito cells in fibrotic livers of rats treated with chronic carbon tetrachloride administration [35]. The promoter gene for COL1A2 isolated from CFSC-2G was found to be the same from Ito cells of normal rat liver, and regulated by TGF-β under paracrine form. On the other hand, the promoter region of CFSC-5H was clarified to be the same as activated Ito cells (myofibroblast-like cells) and regulated by TGF-β under autocrine form. CFSC-5H expressed a significantly higher level of the COL1A2 mRNA than CFSC-2G dose. Very recently, Inagaki developed both new strains of transgenic mice transfected with COL1A2 mRNA and transfected with CFSC-2G, and found that the gene expression of COL1A2 was increased three times and 17 times in nonparenchymal cells fraction isolated from untreated transgenic mice and carbon tetrachloride-treated transgenic mice with fibrotic liver, respectively. This developed experimental model was able to measure the promoter activity of COL1A2 gene in the process of experimental hepatic fibrosis induced by chronic carbon tetrachloride treatment differentiated from the activity in the process of liver regeneration [36].

Role of matrix metalloproteinase-1 (MMP-1) in recovery from liver fibrosis

Mammalian collagenase in the liver reported by authors in 1974 [11] is now referred to as interstitial collagenase or MMP-1. At present, 17th MMPs are grouped into four subclasses, structurally and functionally [37]. The activity is regulated by several mechanisms, which include regulation of gene expression by cytokines or hormones, extracellular cleavage of proenzyme to active enzyme and specific inhibition of active enzyme by endogenous proteins known as TIMPs. Interstitial collagenase can degrade type I, type III and type X collagens, but cannot degrade other types of collagen such as type IV, type V and type IV, and other components of extracellular matrix such as proteoglycans and glycoproteins. Other MMPs, except MMP-1, MMP-8 and MMP-13, however, cannot degrade type I collagen which is very stable, and there is net deposition of type I collagen in progressive hepatic fibrosis [4–6,9]. Therefore, gene expression of interstitial collagenase in fibrous liver should be important from the standpoint of amelioration of liver fibrosis.

The authors prepared the monolayer culture of fibroblasts derived from rabbit liver in order to clarify the mechanism of interstitial collagenase production by cells obtained from liver [17,18]. Elucidation of the mechanism for MMP-1 gene expression in liver cirrhosis may enable us to develop a new strategy for the treatment of liver cirrhosis. The difference in the mechanisms of MMP-1 production among fibroblasts derived from synovium, gastric mucosa and liver were observed in the same rabbit. All fibroblasts used in this experiment were the fourth-passaged cells in order to exclude macrophages and to obtain uniform cell lines. Synovial fibroblasts secreted a low level of MMP-1 proteins without any treatment and cells treated with PMA (phorbol myristate acetate) produced high levels of MMP-1. Gastric mucosal fibroblasts produced high levels of MMP-1 without any treatment. After treatment of the cells with PMA, MMP-1 production was dramatically increased. Liver fibroblasts did not produce MMP-1 even with PMA treatment [18].

The authors succeeded in inducing MMP-1 production by coculture of fibroblasts and hepatocytes at the cell:number ratio of 3:1. After a long latent period remarkably high-level production of MMP-1 was observed [17]. This abundant quantity of MMP-1 production by fibroblasts contributed to massive necrosis or tissue breakdown in vivo.

Recently the authors observed the gene expression of interstitial collagenase in CCl_4-treated rat liver by reverse transcription-polymerase chain reaction (RT-PCR) and in situ hybridization (submitted). In normal rats, no signals for interstitial collagenase mRNA were observed in the liver by in situ hybridization. In rats with fatty change induced by treatment with CCl_4 for 4 weeks, positive signals for interstitial collagenase mRNA were observed in scattered Ito cells which were identified as α-smooth muscle actin positive cells. In rats treated for 8 weeks, an intensive signal for interstitial collagenase mRNA was observed in several kinds of cells within lobules. On the other hand, cirrhotic liver in rats treated for 12 weeks revealed weak expression of interstitial collagenase mRNA in Ito cells. RT-PCR analysis also revealed gene expression of interstitial collagenase in rats treated for 8 weeks. No hepatocytes in the liver displayed interstitial collagenase mRNA transcripts, regardless of CCl_4 treatment. Thus, the authors observed positive signals in activated Ito cells. Activated Ito cells can produce matrix components as well as MMP-1, as reported by Iredale et al. in autoimmune chronic active hepatitis [38]. Their results suggested that Ito cells produce MMP-1 to accumulate fibrosis. There is no paper to demonstrate MMP-1 production by Ito cells in a process of hepatic fibrolysis. Recently, the authors pointed out the evidence of participation of interstitial collagenase to destroy matrix in the recovery stage of hepatic fibrosis. The aim of the present study is to elucidate the gene expression of interstitial collagenase in the recovery stage of experimental rat liver fibrosis.

28

Generally speaking, as mentioned above, gene expression of interstitial collagenase is weak in the process of rat hepatic fibrogenesis induced by chronic CCl_4 intoxication. On the contrary, in the recovery stage of hepatic fibrosis, very strong expression of interstitial collagenase mRNA was observed in Ito cells as well as in hepatocytes. Intense signals were seen in Ito cells within or alongside resolving fibrous bands and neighboring hepatocytes, especially at the front of resorption. These results indicate the participation of interstitial collagenase expressed in hepatocytes and Ito cells for the matrix degradation during the recovery stage of experimental rat liver fibrosis (paper in preparation).

Role of MMP-2, MMP-3, MT1-MMP, other MMPs and TIMPs in recovery from liver fibrosis

MMP-2, MMP-3, MT1-MMP and other MMPs

Arthur et al. reported that Ito cells secreted a neutral metalloproteinase, 72-kDa type IV collagenase/gelatinase (MMP-2) which can degrade type IV collagen (a component of basement membrane) [39,40]. MMP-2 gene expression is upregulated by TGFβ 1 while MMP-1 gene expression is downregulated by τGFβ. Takahara et al. [41] reported the MMP-2 gene expression is increased in the process of experimental hepatic fibrosis and decreased in liver cirrhosis. In the recovery stage from experimental hepatic fibrosis, gene expression of MMP-2 was shown to be increased on the 3rd and the 7th day after the discontinuation of treatment and decreased on the 14th day. The destruction of pericellular fibrosis may occur very early on in the recovery stage.

In situ hybridization of MMP-2 [42] revealed that vimentin-positive, CD-68 negative mesenchymal cells, which should be Ito cells, showed high transcript levels of τGFβ as well as MMP-2. They observed these gene expressions in the process of hepatic fibrosis in chronic hepatitis. Very recently, Takahara et al. [43] demonstrated that there was dual expression of MMP-2 and MT1-MMP in chronic hepatitis and cirrhosis, and that cytoplasmic and membranous immunodeposits of both MMPs were found in endothelial cells, Kupffer cells, capillary endothelial cells and lymphocytes. In particular, they observed overexpression of MMPs in Ito cells and fibroblasts, and suggested that MT1-MMP activates pro-MMP-2 and activates MMP-2 to remodel liver parenchyma during the process of liver fibrosis. It has been found that gene expression of MMP-2 increases in the liver fibrosis and decreases in cirrhosis [41]. MMP-2 expression is stimulated by TGF-β. The behavior of gene expression is very different between interstitial collagenase and MMP-2. The authors presume that MMP-2 does not contribute to the recovery, since MMP-2 gene expression has not been observed during the process of fibrolysis in the liver by in situ hybridization.

Vyas et al. [44] reported that cultured rat Ito cells synthesized and secreted transin (stromelysin). Herbst et al. [45] revealed that gene expression of MMP-3 in hepatocytes was observed during the early phase of rat liver regeneration after a single injection of CCl_4. At the site of this gene expression, both c-fos and c-jun transcripts were also observed by in situ hybridization. Winwood et al. [46] reported that Kupffer cells secreted 95-kd type IV collagenase/gelatinase B. MMP-3 and MMP-9 should be investigated by more a specific technique in relation to perihepatocellular fibrosis. MMP-3 gene expression has not been observed during the process of fibrolysis in hepatic fibrosis. Gene expression of MT1-MMP and other MMPs has not been studied during the process of fibrolysis in the liver.

TIMPs

The metabolism of extracellular matrix is regulated with 17 MMPs in cooperated with their specific TIMP-1, -2, -3, and -4 [47—51]. Iredale et al. [48] and Roeb et al. [49] demonstrated that TIMP-1 mRNA expression was increased during the early phase of CCl_4 treatment and subsequently decreased and stayed at a low level during the experiment. Net activity of MMPs is determined by the balance between activities of MMPs and their inhibitors. Herbst et al. [50] revealed that TIMP-1 and TIMP-2 transcripts were present predominantly in Ito cells at high levels in both fibrotic rat and human livers. However, TIMPs have not been examined during the recovery phase of experimental hepatic fibrosis.

Serum levels of MMPs and TIMPs

The authors measured the serum levels of MMPs in patients with chronic hepatitis C and compared the levels before treatment with those after interferon therapy in relation to the improvement of liver fibrosis [22]. Table 1 shows that serum level of MMP-1 and/or TIMPs increase in responder patients. Table 2 indicates the ratio of MMP-1:TIMP-1 or -2, which increases after interferon therapy. These data suggest that serum level of MMP-1 or the ratio of MMP-1:TIMP-1 (or -2) is a good indicator showing matrix degradation in liver fibrosis.

Conclusion

Table 1. Number of cases with increased serum MMPs and TIMPs levels after interferon treatment.

	Responders (n = 7)		Nonresponders (n = 11)		χ^2test p^a
	↑	→/↓	↑	→/↓	
MMP-1	5	2	0	11	< 0.01
MMP-2	3	4	5	6	n.s.
MMP-3	2	5	4	7	n.s.
TIMP-1	5	2	1	10	< 0.05
TIMP-2	3	4	8	3	n.s.

[a]Statistical significance was tested by χ^2 test.

Table 2. Number of cases with increased MMPs:TIMPs ratios after interferon treatment.

	Responders (n = 7)		Nonresponders (n = 11)		χ^2 test p^a
	↑	→/↓	↑	→/↓	
MMP-1/TIMP-1	6	1	0	11	< 0.005
MMP-2/TIMP-1	3	4	2	9	n.s.
MMP-3/TIMP-1	4	3	2	9	n.s.
MMP-1/TIMP-2	5	2	1	10	< 0.05
MMP-2/TIMP-2	4	3	7	4	n.s.
MMP-3/TIMP-2	2	5	8	6	n.s.

[a]Statistical significance was tested by χ^2 test (see [22]).

Laminin, interferons, cAMP-related compounds, methylxanthines, FK506, L-nitro-arginine, and retinylester have been found to inhibit the activation of Ito cells. Since the authors believe that interstitial collagenase may destroy fibrous tissue and contribute to the recovery from liver fibrosis, the regulation of interstitial collagenase gene expression should be a key step towards curing liver fibrosis. On the other hand, the incidence of hepatocellular carcinoma may possibly be induced by constitutive gene expression of interstitial collagenase from the findings of the transient gene expression of interstitial collagenase in very early hepatocellular carcinoma (less than 2 cm in diameter) [23]. The possibility of the clinical usage of this enzyme makes us excited, although careful observations should be made for further study.

References

1. Bissell DM. Cell-matrix interaction and hepatic fibrosis. In: Popper H, Schaffner F (eds) Progress in Liver Diseases 9. Philadelphia, New York: Grune & Stratton Inc., 1990;143—155.
2. Friedman SL. Seminars in medicine of the Beth Israel Hospital, Boston. The cellular basis of hepatic fibrosis. Mechanisms and treatment strategies. N Engl J Med 1993;328:1828—1835.
3. Friedman SL. Molecular mechanisms of hepatic fibrosis and principles of therapy. J Gastroenterol 1997;32:424—430.
4. Bissell DM. Connective tissue metabolism and hepatic fibrosisan overview. Sem Liv Dis 1990; 10:3—14.
5. Arthur MJP. Matrix degradation in the liver. Sem Liv Dis 1990;10:47—55.
6. Arthur MJP. Role of Ito cells in the degradation of matrix in liver. J Gastroenterol Hepatol 1995;10:557—562.
7. Rubin E, Hutterer F. Hepatic fibrosis: studies in the formation and resorption. In: Wagner BM, Smith DE (eds) The Connective Tissue. Baltimore: Williams and Wilkins Co., 1967;142—160.
8. Perez-Tamayo R. Some aspects of connective tissue of the liver. In: Popper H, Schaffner F (eds) Progress in Liver Diseases 2. Philadelphia, New York: Grune & Stratton Inc., 1965;192—210.
9. Rojkind M, Dunn MA. Hepatic fibrosis. Gastroenterology 1979;76:849—863.
10. Cameron GR, Karunaratne WAE. Carbon tetrachloride cirrhosis in relation to liver regeneration. J Pathol Bacterial 1936;42:1—21.
11. Okazaki I, Maruyama K. Collagenase activity in experimental hepatic fibrosis. Nature 1974; 252:49—50.

12. Maruyama K, Feinman L, Okazaki I, Lieber CS. Direct measurement of neutral collagenase activity in homogenates from baboon and human liver. Biochem Biophys Acta 1981;658: 124–131.

13. Maruyama K, Okazaki I, Kashiwazaki K, Miyairi M, Oda M, Ishii H, Tsuchiya M. A case of subacute hepatitis with reversible liver fibrosis. Gastroenterol Jpn 1981;16:611–615.

14. Okazaki I, Brinckerhoff CE, Sinclair JR, Sinclair PR, Bonkowsky HL, Harris ED Jr. Iron increases collagenase production by rabbit synovial fibroblasts. J Lab Clin Med 1981;97: 396–402.

15. Maruyama K, Feinman L, Fainsilber Z, Nakano M, Okazaki I, Lieber CS. Mammalian collagenase increases in early alcoholic liver disease and decreases with cirrhosis. Life Sci 1982; 30:1379–1384.

16. Okazaki I, Feinman L, Fainsilber Z, Nakano M, Lieber CS. Development of an assay for hepatic mammalian collagenase and study of the effect of ethanol on enzyme activity. In: Lieber CS (ed) Biological Approach to Alcoholism. Rockville, Maryland, USA: Public Health, 1983; 392–398.

17. Maruyama K, Okazaki I, Kobayashi T, Suzuki H, Kashiwazaki K, Tsuchiya M. Collagenase production by rabbit liver cells in monolayer culture. J Lab Clin Med 1983;102:543–550.

18. Okazaki I, Maruyama K, Kashiwazaki K, Tsuchiya M. Mechanism of collagenase production by liver cells. In: Hirayama C, Kivirikko KI (eds) Pathobiology of Hepatic Fibrosis. Amsterdam: Elsevier Science Publishers 1985;141–149.

19. Okazaki I, Maruyama K, Kashiwazaki K, Ebihara Y, Shigeta Y, Ishii H, Tsuchiya M. Type-specific collagen-degrading enzyme activity in alcoholic liver disease. In: Kamada T, Kuriyama K, Suwaki H (eds) Biomedical Aspects of Alcohol and Alcoholism. Tokyo: Gendaikikakushitu Publishers, 1988;329–339.

20. Maruyama K, Okazaki I, Kashiwazaki K, Sonoda I, Ishii H, Tsuchiya M, Shibata T, Inayama S. Biosynthesis of Type IV collagenase by hepatic sinusoidal cells in rats. Acta Hepatol Jpn 1987; 28:973–974.

21. Maruyama K, Okazaki I, Takagi T, Ishii, H. Formation and degradation of basement membrane collagen. Alcohol Alcoholism 1991;26(Suppl 1):309–374.

22. Arai M, Niioka M, Maruyama K, Wada N, Fujimoto N, Nomiyama T, Tanaka S, Okazaki I. Changes in serum levels of metalloproteinases and their inhibitors by treatment of chronic hepatitis C with interferon. Dig Dis Sci 1996;41:995–1000.

23. Okazaki I, Wada N, Nakano M, Saito A, Takasaki K, Doi M, Kameyama K, Otani Y, Kubochi K, Niioka M, Watanabe T, Maruyama K. Difference in gene expression for matrix metalloproteinase-1 between early and advanced hepatocellular carcinomas. Hepatology 1997;25: 580–584.

24. Takahara, Kojima T, Miyabayashi C, Inoue K, Sasaki H, Muragaki Y, Ooshima A. Collagen production in fat-storing cells after carbon tetrachloride intoxication in the rat. Immunoelectron microscopic observation of type I, type III collagens, and prolyl hydroxylase. Lab Invest 1988; 50:509–521.

25. Milani S, Herbst H, Schuppan D, Hahn EG, Stein H. In situ hybridization for procollagen types I, III and IV mRNA in normal and fibrotic rat liver: evidence for predominant expression in nonparenchymal liver cells. Hepatology 1989;10:84–92.

26. Armendariz-Borunda J, Seyer JM, Kang AH, Raghow R. Regulation of TGFβ gene expression in rat liver intoxicated with carbon tetrachloride. FASEB J 1990;4:215–221.

27. Lee KS, Buck M, Houglum K, Chojkier M. Activation of hepatic stellate cells by TGF-β and collagen type I is mediated by oxidative stress through c-myb expression. J Clin Invest 1995; 96:2461–2468.

28. Weiner FR, Blaner WS, Czaja MJ, Shah A, Geerts A. Ito cell expression of a nuclear retinoic acid receptor. Hepatology 1992;15:336–342.

29. Okuno M, Moriwaki H, Imai S, Muto Y, Kawada N, Suzuki Y, Kojima S. Retinoids exacerbate rat liver fibrosis by inducing the activation of latent TGF-β in liver stellate cells. Hepatology

1997;26:913—921.
30. Rockey DC, Chung JJ. Endothelin antagonism in experimental hepatic fibrosis. J Clin Invest 1996;98:1381—1388.
31. Pinzani M, Marra F, Caligiuri A, DeFranco R, Gentilini A, Failli P, Gentilini P. Inhibition by pentoxifylline of extracellular signal-regulated kinase activation by platelet-derived growth factor in hepatic stellate cells. Br J Pharmacol 1996;119:1117—1124.
32. Marra F, Gentilini A, Pinzani M, Choudhury GG, Parola M, Herbst H, Dianzani MU, Laffi G, Abboud HE, Gentilini P. Phosphatidylinositol 3-kinase is required for platelet-derived growth factor's action on hepatic stellate cells. Gastroenterol 1997;112:1297—1306.
33. Inagaki Y, Truter S, Ramirez F. Transforming growth factor-β stimulates α2(1) collagen gene expression through a cis-acting element that contains an Sp1-binding site. J Biol Chem 1994; 269:14828—14834.
34. Inagaki Y, Truter S, Tanaka S, Di Liberto M, Ramirez F. Overlapping pathways mediate the opposing actions of tumor necrosis factor-β and transforming growth factor-β on α2(1) collagen gene transcription. J Biol Chem 1995;270:3353—3358.
35. Inagaki Y, Truter S, Greenwel P, Rojkind M, Unoura M, Kobayashi K, Ramirez F. Regulation of the α2(1) collagen gene transcription in fat-storing cells derived from a cirrhotic liver. Hepatology 1995;22:573—579.
36. Inagaki Y, Nemoto T. Luciferase quantitative assay for promoter gene activity of COL1A2. Acta Hepatol Jpn 1998;30(Suppl 1):172 (Abstract).
37. Nagase H, Barret A, Woessner J. Nomenclature and glossary of the matrix metalloproteinases. Matrix 1992;1(Suppl):421—424.
38. Iredale J, Goddard S, Murphy G, Benyon R, Arthur M. Tissue inhibitor of metalloproteinase-1 and interstitial collagenase expression in autoimmune chronic active hepatitis and activated human hepatic lipocytes. Clin Sci 1995;89:75—81.
39. Arthur M, Friedman S, Roll F, Bissell D. Lipocytes from normal rat liver release a neutral metalloproteinase that degrades basement membrane (type IV) collagen. J Clin Inv 1989;84: 1076—1085.
40. Arthur M, Stanley A, Iredale J, Rafferty J, Hembry R, Friedman S. Secretion of 72 kDa type IV collagenase/gelatinase by cultured human lipocytes. Biochem J 1992;287:701—707.
41. Takahara T, Furui K, Funaki J et al. Increased expression of matrix metalloproteinase-II in experimental liver fibrosis in rats. Hepatology 1995;21:787—795.
42. Milani S, Herbst H, Schuppan D, Grappone C, Pellegrini G, Pinzani M et al. Differential expression of matrix-metalloproteinase-1 and -2 genes in normal and fibrotic human liver. Am J Pathol 1994;144:528—537.
43. Takahara T, Furui K, Yata Y, Jin B, Zhang LP, Nanbu S, Sato H, Seiki M, Watanabe A. Dual expression of matrix metalloproteinase-2 and membrane-type 1-matrix metalloproteinase in fibrotic human livers. Hepatology 1997;26:1521—1529.
44. Vyas SK, Leyland H, Gentry J, Arthur MJP. Rat hepatic lipocytes synthesize and secrete transin (stromelysin) in early primary culture. Gastroenterol 1995;109:889—898.
45. Herbst H, Heinrichs O, Schuppan D, Milani S, Stein H. Temporal and spatial patterns of transin/stromelysin RNA expression following toxic injury in rat liver. Virchows Archiv B Cell Pathol 1991;60:295—300.
46. Winwood PJ, Schuppan D, Iredale JP, Kawser CA, Docherty AJP, Arthur MJP. Kupffer cell-derived 95-kd type IV collagenase/gelatinase B: characterization and expression in cultured cells. Hepatology 1995;22:304—315.
47. Iredale JP, Murphy G, Hembry RM, Friedman SL, Arthur MJ. Human hepatic lipocytes synthesize tissue inhibitor of metalloproteinases-1. J Clin Invest 1992;90:282—287.
48. Iredale J, Benyon R, Arthur M, Ferris W, Alcolado R, Winwood P et al. Tissue inhibitor of metalloproteinase-1 messenger RNA expression is enhanced relative to interstitial collagenase messenger RNA in experimental liver injury and fibrosis. Hepatology 1996;24:176—184.
49. Roeb E, Purucker E, Breuer B, Nguyen H, Heinrich PC, Rose-John S et al. TIMP expression in

toxic and cholestatic liver injury in rat. J Hepatology 1997;27:535–544.
50. Herbst H, Wege T, Milani S et al. Tissue inhibitor of metalloproteinase-1 and -2 RNA expression in rat and human liver fibrosis. Am J Pathol 1997;150:1647–1659.
51. Iredale JP. Tissue inhibitors of metalloproteinases in liver fibrosis. Int J Cell Biol 1997;29: 43–54.

Progress in Hepatology, Volume 4.
Liver Cirrhosis Update.
M. Yamanaka et al., editors.

35

Inflammation: mediated hepatocarcinogenesis — hypercarcinogenic state of chronic liver disease

Okio Hino, Toshiki Yamamoto and Kazunori Kajino
Department of Experimental Pathology, Cancer Institute, Tokyo, Japan

Abstract. Hepatitis viral, "inflammation mediated" hepatocarcinogenesis greatly influences the incidence of somatic genetic events in hepatocytes, by increasing the number of target cells, or the proliferation of once-hit hepatocytes, eventually leading to hepatocellular carcinomas (HCCs). These conditions may be designated as the "hypercarcinogenic state". Our goal is to lead the "hypocarcinogenic state" to the "normo- or hypocarcinogenic" state and to prevent HCC development.

Keywords: hepatocarcinogenesis, hepatocellular carcinoma, hypercarcinogenic state.

Introduction

Persistent hepatitis B virus (HBV)/hepatitis C virus (HCV) infection is epidemiologically closely associated with the development of human hepatocellular carcinoma (HCC). Among HBV/HCV carriers, HCC usually develops in patients with chronic liver disease, such as chronic active hepatitis or cirrhosis. In other words, a hepatitis-related proliferative change, which is mainly sustained by repeated cycles of cell death and regeneration, appears to be important for HBV/HCV hepatocarcinogenesis. The accumulation of mutations, which are likely to occur during continuous cycles of cell division, may eventually transform some hepatocytes through a multistage process. The question of whether HBV or HCV themselves act as carcinogenic factors, independent of any hepatitis-related proliferative change, however, is still being debated.

Since 1975, the number of hepatocellular carcinoma (HCC) patients has been increasing in Japan. In 1995, 30,000 people were killed by HCC, and it was the third leading cause of death in the malignancy [1]. Most HCCs occurred in the patients infected with HBV or HCV. Recently, we have succeeded in diminishing HBV carriers and HBV-associated liver diseases by the HBV vaccination to prevent vertical infection, and by the exclusion of HBsAg carriers from blood donors. On the contrary, the amount of HCV-associated liver disease has been increasing in those who had received the blood transfusion containing HCV before the establishment of HCV screening system in Japan. Thus the number of HBV and HCV carriers are still estimated to be 2—4 million in Japan. Other

Address for correspondence: Okio Hino MD, PhD, Department of Experimental Pathology, Cancer Institute, 1-37-1 Kami-Ikebukuro, Toshima-ku, Tokyo 170-8455, Japan. Tel.: +81-3-5394-3815. Fax: +81-3-5394-3815. E-mail: ohino@ims.u-tokyo.ac.jp.

than the interferon treatment, an effective therapy for HBV and HCV infection has not yet been established, and in the future, more patients may suffer from chronic liver disease and HCC. The prevalence of chronic liver disease is a serious public problem in Japan. To solve this problem, we must understand the molecular mechanism of hepatitis and hepatocarcinogenesis.

In Table 1, we show the etiology of HCC. In Japan, 70–80% of HCC is caused by HCV infection, and 10–20% by HBV infection (Fig. 1). HCC of unknown etiology still exists and accounts for several percent. Some groups reported that integrated HBV DNA is found in HBsAg-negative HCC patients at a very high frequency and that HBV might have a more ubiquitous causal role for HCCs than was previously considered [2]. However, in our study by Southern blotting, only three of 44 HBsAg-negative HCC patients were found to have the HBV integration [3]. We consider that the causative role of HBV is not significant for HBsAg-negative HCCs in Japan.

The natural history of HBV and HCV carriers is shown in Fig. 2. From the clinical aspect, there are some differences in the history between patients infected with two viruses. A few cases of HBV-associated HCC occurred in young patients, and in these cases, the integration of HBV DNA may have induced HCC directly. Most patients with HBV- and HCV-associated liver diseases develop HCC after a 20–30 year history of chronic hepatitis or liver cirrhosis. The background liver condition is shown in Fig. 3. This means the progression from asymptomatic carrier to the chronic hepatitis may be the first step of hepatocaricinogenesis. Most HBV-carriers are infected in their childhood and about 10% of HBV-carriers develop chronic hepatitis. Most HCV carriers are infected by a blood transfusion or needle. Compared with HBV carriers, fewer patients can clear the virus infection naturally, and about 60–80% of them develop chronic hepatitis. We estimate that about 20% of HCV carriers develop HCC, while the incidence of HCC in HBV carriers is about 5%.

In patients with HBV-associated HCC, integrated HBV DNA has been detected in approximately 90% of HCC tissues [4]. From the analysis of the HBV integration modes, it has been reported that the integration sites are random in the host genomic DNA, indicating that the HBV integration mode is peculiar to each HCC case [5]. The integration is considered to occur before or at the initial stage of neoplastic proliferation, and, therefore, many studies used

Table 1. Causes of HCCs.

Hepatitis viruses (HBV, HCV)
Alcohol
Afratoxin
Autoimmune diseases (PBC, primary biliary cirrhosis; AIH, autoimmune hepatitis)
Metabolic diseases (hemochromatosis, Wilson's disease)
Drugs (oral contraception drug, anabolic steroid)
Budd-Chiari syndrome
Unknown

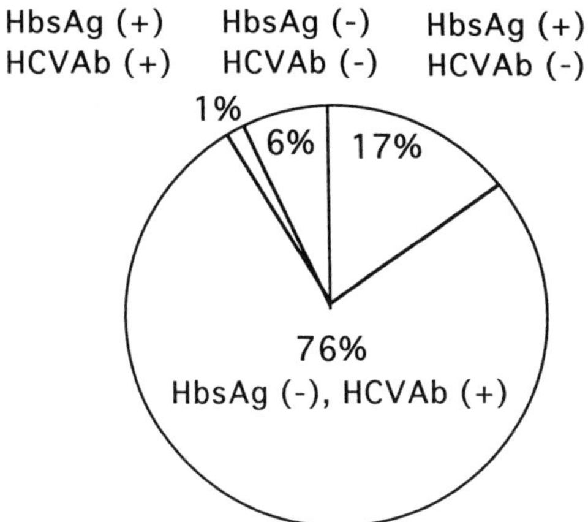

Fig. 1. Causative agents of HCC.

the integration pattern as the marker of the clonality of HCC. For example, several groups reported that in most of the advanced multiple HCC cases, each tumor showed the identical HBV integration pattern, indicating that the multiple HCCs are caused by the intrahepatic metastasis [6—8]. On the other hand, in cases having more than two small HCCs, the modes of HBV integration were different between tumors [9,10]. This means that advanced HCC has the ability of

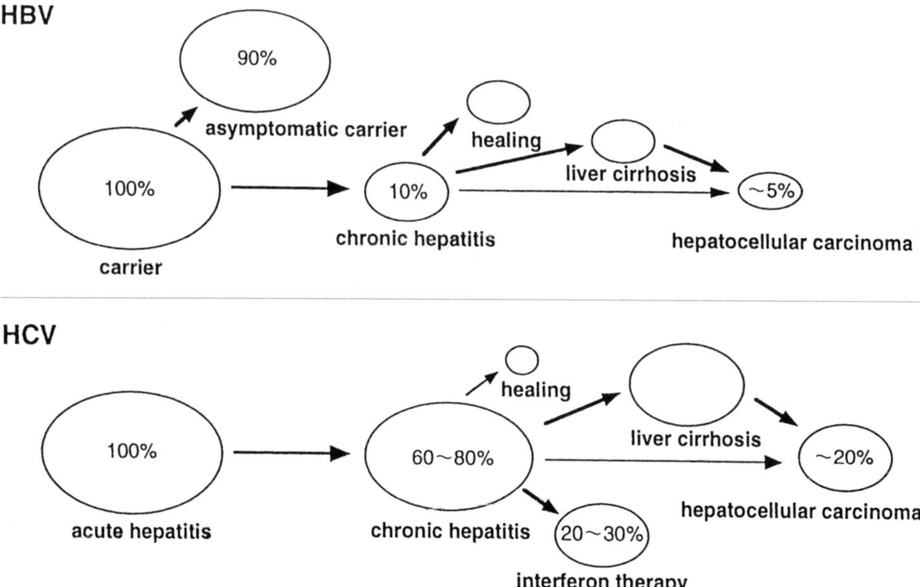

Fig. 2. Natural history of HBV and HCV carriers.

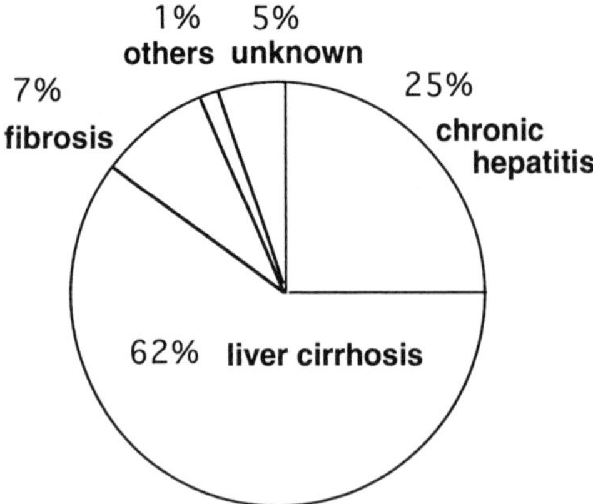

Fig. 3. Background liver conditions of HCC.

metastasis in the progression and dissemination of the multiple loci in the liver, and that in the early HCC cases, they were more likely to be the result of multi-centric occurrence, probably because each tumor does not have the characteristics of metastasis.

The recurrence rate of HCC after a curative operation is 20–40% in 1 year and about 80% in 5 years in Japan, and these rates are higher than other solitary tumors. In spite of technical advances in the treatment and early detection, long-time survival rate has not improved. All these data support the contention that liver cirrhosis is the state of "Field cancarization" where the multiple HCCs are likely to occur [11]. This concept of "Field cancarization" also reflects the situation where multiple genetic mutations easily occur and accumulate, and this may also be called a "hypercarcinogenic state" [12]. Yasui et al. reported on the HBV integration modes with the regenerative nodules in the liver cirrhosis patients [13]. They studied a total of 83 cirrhotic nodules from 11 cirrhotic livers of HBV-carrier patients using Southern blotting. According to their report, integrated HBV DNA was shown in 26 of 83 nodules and 0–74% variation existed in the positive rates for integration in nodules among livers. These nodules with the HBV integration did not have any neoplastic-appearing foci in nodules, despite the fact that the detection sensitivity would predict clones of more than 10^5 cells to give rise to clonal integration patterns on Southern blotting. As the technical advancement for small HCC treatments reaches a sufficient level, we must try to change the hypercarcinogenic to normo- or hypocarcinogenic state, and prevent the occurrence of HCC at the cirrhosis stage to improve the prognosis of chronic liver diseases.

Conclusion

We propose that the hepatitis virus can cause an increase in the incidence of HCC by a combination of two mechanisms:

i) cell killing and stimulation of mitosis leading to an accumulation of events necessary for transformation, and

ii) an increase in chromosomal instability mediated by induced recombinogenic protein(s) during chronic hepatitis [14,15].

References

1. Health and Welfare Statistics Association. Health and Welfare Statistics in Japan. Japan: J Health Welfare Atat Chapt 2, 1997;60—61.

2. Bréchot C, Degos F, Lugassy C, Thiers V, Zafrani S, Franco D, Bismuth H, Trépo D, Benhamou J-P, Wands J, Isselbacher K, Tiollais P, Berthelot P. Hepatitis B virus DNA in patients with chronic liver disease and negative tests for hepatitis B surface antigen. N Engl J Med 1985;312: 270—276.

3. Hino O, Kitagawa T, Sugano H. Relationship between serum and histochemical markers for hepatitis B virus and rate of viral integration in hepatocellular carcinomas in Japan. Int J Cancer 1985;35:5—10.

4. Hino O, Ohtake K, Rogler CE. Features of two hepatitis B virus (HBV) DNA integrations suggest mechanisms of HBV integration. J Virol 1989;63:2638—2543.

5. Matsubara K, Tokino T. Integration of hepatitis B virus DNA and its implications for hepatocarcinogenesis. Molec Biol Med 1990;7:243—260.

6. Esumi M, Arikata T, Arii M, Suzuki K, Tanikawa K, Mizuo H, Mima T, Shikata T. Clonal origin of human hepatoma determined by integration of hepatitis B virus DNA. Cancer Res 1986;46:5767—5771.

7. Imazeki F, Omata M, Yokosuka O, Okuda K. Integration of hepatitis B virus DNA in hepatocellular carcinoma. Cancer 1986;58:1055—1060.

8. Govindarajan S, Craig JR, Valinluck B. Clonal origin of hepatitis B virus-associated hepatocellular carcinoma. Hum Pathol 1988;19:403—405.

9. Hsu HC, Chiou TJ, Chen JY, Lee CS, Lee PH, Pen SY. Clonality and clonal evolution of hepatocellular carcinoma with multiple nodules. Hepatology 1991;13:923—928.

10. Sheu JC, Huang GT, Chou HC, Lee PH, Wang JT, Lee HS, Chen DS. Multiple hepatocellular carcinomas at the early stage have different clonality. Gastroenterology 1993;105:1471—1476.

11. Slaughter DP, Southwick HW, Smejkal W. Field cancerization in oral stratified squamous epithelium: clinical implications of multicentric origins. Cancer 1953;5:963—968.

12. Hino O. Preface: mechanisms of viral carcinogenesis; from hypercarcinogenic to normo- or hypocarcinogenic states. Intervirology 1995;38:125—126.

13. Yasui H, Hino O, Ohtake K, Machinami R, Kitagawa T. Clonal growth of hepatitis B virus-integrated hepatocytes in cirrhotic liver nodules. Cancer Res 1992;52:6810—6814.

14. Hino O, Tabata S, Hotta Y. Evidence for increased in vitro recombination with insertion of human hepatitis B virus DNA Proc Natl Acad Sci USA 1991;88:9248—9252.

15. Aoki H, Kajino K, Arakawa Y, Hino O. Molecular cloning of a rat chromosome putative recombinogenic sequence homologous to the hepatitis B virus encasidation signal. Proc Natl Acad Sci USA 1996;93:7300—7304.

Progress in Hepatology, Volume 4.
Liver Cirrhosis Update.
M. Yamanaka et al., editors.

41

Imaging diagnosis of portal hypertension

Shoichi Matsutani and Hiromitsu Saisho
First Department of Medicine, Chiba University School of Medicine, Chiba, Japan

Abstract. Imaging diagnosis is now widely used in the clinical practice of portal hypertension. Among several noninvasive modalities, ultrasound alone, or with Doppler examination, is the most important as a first step to assess patients. The presence of splenomegaly or portosystemic collaterals and the causes of portal hypertension can be evaluated noninvasively by these technologies. The assessment of the blood flow in portosystemic collaterals using Doppler flowmetry may help to evaluate the hemodynamic grade of gastroesophageal varices. Angiography has been up until now a golden standard with which to diagnose abnormal vasculature in portal hypertension. However, computed tomography (CT) or magnetic resonance imaging will replace angiography to assess them in the near future. Noninvasive imaging diagnosis will be the most important in the assessment and management of patients with portal hypertension.

Keywords: noninvasive imaging, portal hemodynamics, portosystemic collaterals.

Introduction

Imaging diagnosis is now widely used to assess the clinical manifestations and the causes of portal hypertension [1–2]. Furthermore, recent advances in imaging technologies have made it possible to diagnose portal hypertension more conveniently and noninvasively. In the clinical practice of portal hypertension, the methods used as a first-step approach to assess the patients are ultrasonography, Doppler flowmetry or color Doppler and endoscopy. Ultrasonography (US) alone or with Doppler examination is important in terms of the financial costs for the patients and the risk of ionizing radiation. Furthermore, these modalities are suitable to evaluate a patient who is in an emergency or critical state such as variceal hemorrhage, which occurs frequently in patients with portal hypertension. Doppler flowmetry and color Doppler can assess the presence, direction and flow velocity of blood flow in the portal vein system, the hepatic vein and the various abdominal arteries. The advantages of these techniques are that they are convenient, noninvasive and allow the real-time evaluation of portal and splanchnic hemodynamics at the bedside of the patients. However, it is necessary to know the potential disadvantages of these techniques that are dependant on the technique of the operator, the limitations created by body habitus and the need to correct the angle of insonation in quantitative analysis. In this chapter, image findings in patients with portal hypertension observed by US, Doppler

---

Address for correspondence: Shoichi Matsutani MD, First Department of Medicine, Chiba University School of Medicine, 1-8-1 Inohana Chuo-ku, Chiba 260, Japan.

flowmetry, color Doppler and computed tomography (CT) are shown and new technologies employed in the imaging diagnosis of portal hypertension are briefly explained.

Diagnosis of splenomegaly

Diagnosis of splenomegaly is important because it is a first step or clue towards the suspicion of the presence of portal hypertension. The upper limits of normal splenic size are a length of 13 cm, an anterior-posterior diameter of 7 cm and a thickness of 4 cm [3]. Imaging diagnosis is helpful in the detection of a slightly enlarged spleen which physical examination cannot demonstrate. The method by which to assess the size of the spleen using US as spleen index is shown in Fig. 1. From the study of normal adults, splenomegaly is diagnosed, by US, by an index score greater than 20 cm [4]. In the assessment of spleen size by CT, splenomegaly is defined as a longitudinal length greater than 15 cm by and is calculated by the number of image slices including the spleen. Imaging diagnosis is also helpful when trying to observe the changes in the size of the spleen during the natural course or the course after treatment of portal hypertension. Spleno-megaly and hypersplenism are good signs by which to suspect the presence of portal hypertension. However, they are not specific to portal hypertension, because they occur in patients with infectious diseases, blood disorders, and many other diseases without portal hypertension. Images of the spleen do not help the differential diagnosis of the causes of splenomegaly. In portal hyperten-sion, the size of the spleen usually does not correlate with portal pressure or the endoscopic grade of gastroesophageal varices. Although hypersplenism is fre-quent in patients having portal hypertension with a markedly enlarged spleen, the size of the spleen does not usually correlate with the grade of hypersplenism.

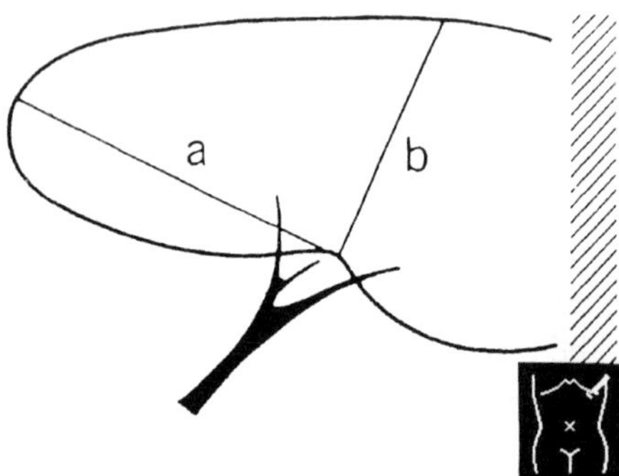

Fig. 1. The methods used to measure the size of the spleen by US. On the section of the largest area of the spleen that contains the splenic hilum, the distance between the hilar indentation and anterior mergin indicated as "a" and the length of the perpendicular to it indicated as "b" are measured. The product of a and b is the spleen index.

Diagnosis of portosystemic collaterals

The diagnosis of portosystemic collaterals is important in the management of patients with portal hypertension because portosystemic collaterals are closely related to the development of gastroesophageal varices and hepatic encephalopathy which are the major complications of portal hypertension. Angiography has been a golden standard in the assessment of portosystemic collaterals [5]. However, now, US, CT and magnetic resonance imaging (MRI) can demonstrate their presence noninvasively. Furthermore, Doppler-US can show and measure the blood flow in a portosystemic collateral conveniently and in real time. Portosystemic collaterals, which can be located by imaging diagnosis, are the paraumbilical vein (PUV), the left gastric vein (LGV), the spleno-renal shunt (SRS) and the mesenteric venous shunt. US and enhanced CT images of these collateral veins are shown in Figs. 2 and 3. Among the portosystemic collaterals, the LGV is the most important because it is the major pathway to the esophageal varices, the bleeding of which is the most serious complication in portal hypertension. Therefore, the assessment of the blood flow in the LGV is important in estimat-

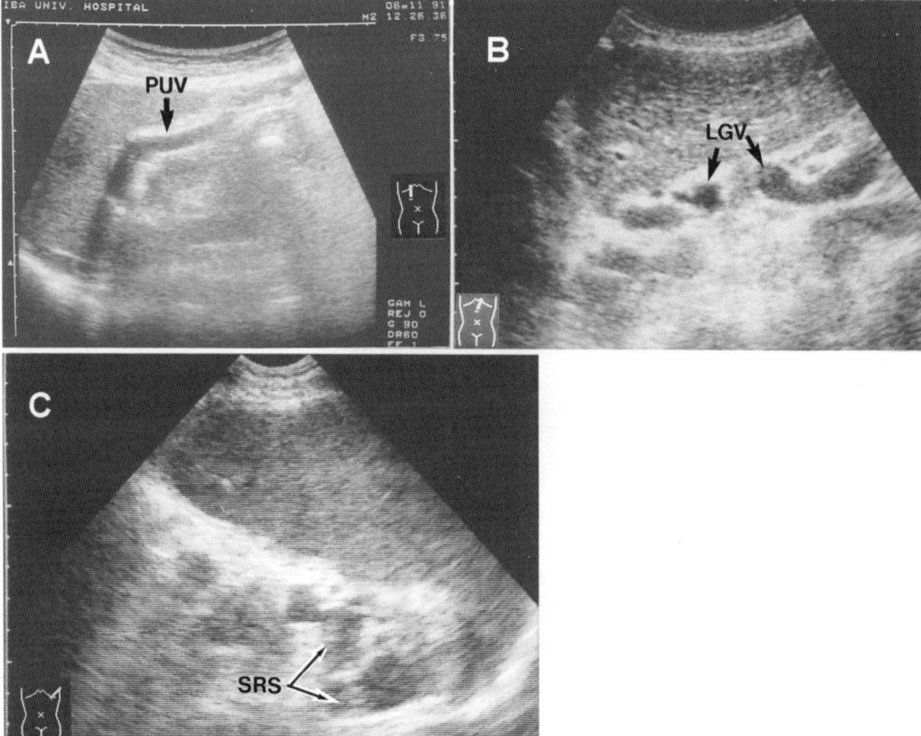

Fig. 2. US images of portosystemic collaterals in portal hypertension. **A**: The paraumbilical vein. **B**: The left gastric vein. **C**: The spleno-renal shunt.

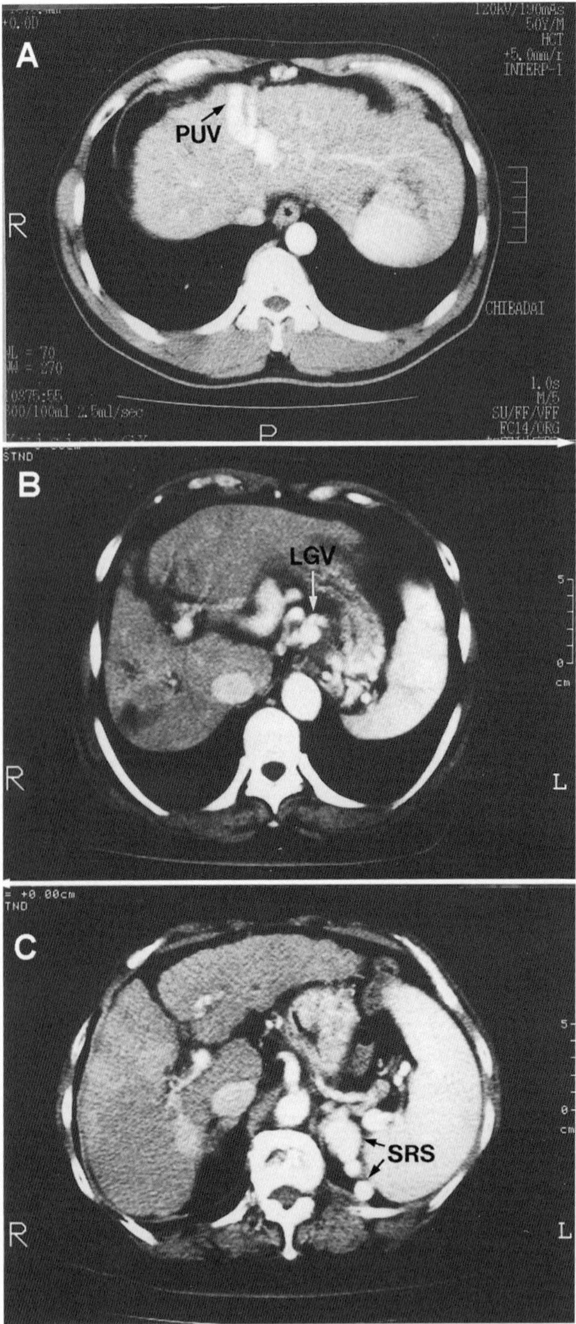

Fig. 3. Enhanced CT images of portosystemic collaterals in portal hypertension. A: The paraumbilical vein. B: The left gastric vein. C: The spleno-renal shunt.

ing, even indirectly, the hemodynamic grade of gastroesophageal varices. In patients with esophageal varices, the LGV is usually enlarged more than 4 mm, and hepatofugal blood flow in the LGV increases as the size of esophageal varices enlarges [4,6]. It has been known from studies by Doppler flowmetry that not only portal flow but also hepatofugal blood flow in the LGV increases rapidly after the intake of a meal (Fig. 4) [6]. An increase in variceal blood flow by vari-

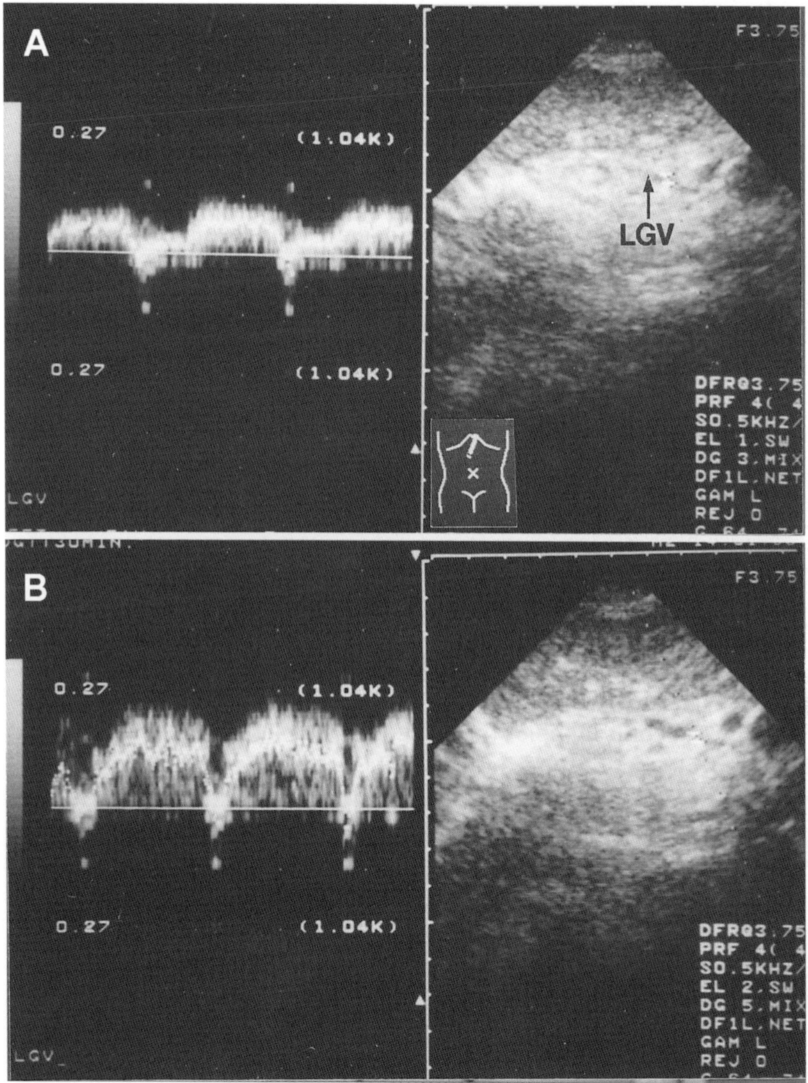

Fig. 4. Changes of blood flow in the left gastric vein after the intake of glucose. **A:** Before glucose intake, hepatofugal blood flow is observed in the left gastric vein. **B:** After glucose intake, an increase of blood flow is observed 30 min after the intake of glucose.

46

ous stimuli, such as a meal or vasoactive substances like glucagon etc., may contribute to the onset of variceal bleeding. Analysis of these hemodynamics in gastroesophageal varices by Doppler-US may be valuable in understanding the mechanism and the risk of variceal hemorrhage. Measurement of the LGV flow is also useful in the assessment of the effect of pharmacotherapy for esophageal varices, using vasopressin or propranolol, which helps to select the responders to the vasoactive drugs [7].

Diagnosis of the cause of portal hypertension

A precise diagnosis of the cause of portal hypertension can help to estimate the prognosis of patients because the clinical course of noncirrhotic portal hypertension is usually good when bleeding from gastroesophageal varices is successfully controlled. US, aided Doppler-US, is valuable in the diagnosis of liver cirrhosis (LC), extrahepatic portal obstruction (EHO), hepatic schistosomiasis and Budd-Chiari syndrome through evaluating the changes in the liver, the portal vein and the hepatic vein. Color Doppler is valuable in detecting portal vein thrombosis by demonstrating the lack of blood flow signals in the portal vein. Color Doppler is also able to diagnose an arterio-portal fistula by demonstrating reversed flow in the portal vein with increased blood flow in the hepatic artery. Early diagnosis of these causes is important for the treatment because they are causes of rapidly progressive gastroesophageal varices or ascites. Characteristic US images of the diseases that cause portal hypertension are shown in Fig. 5.

Recent advances in imaging technology

Recently developed technologies such as power Doppler [8], contrast-enhanced ultrasound [9–10], 3D-CT portography [11–12] and MR angiography [13] are now employed in the imaging diagnosis of portal hypertension. Power Doppler is a new technology in color Doppler that is able to demonstrate a signal intensity of Doppler shifted ultrasound, which allows the detection of slow flow or flow in a deeply seated vessel by employing the increased Doppler gain. Power Doppler is helpful in the diagnosis of hemodynamic abnormalities in the portal vein such as thrombus formation which usually color Doppler cannot show (Fig. 6). Contrast enhanced ultrasound is also one of the alternatives available in diagnostic ultrasound. The intravenous injection of a contrast agent containing microbubbles less than the size of red blood cells can give an enhancement in US and Doppler images, thereby showing fine vasculature images in abdominal organs and vessels. Application of these newly developed ultrasound technologies will help to diagnose abnormal blood flow in the portal hypertensive liver and the portal vein system in more detail. CT or MR portography can demonstrate the portal vein and its tributaries noninvasively and stereologically (Fig. 7). Noninvasive and precise assessment of the gastroesophageal collaterals will be useful in deciding upon therapeutic strategies for the treatment of varices. Though the

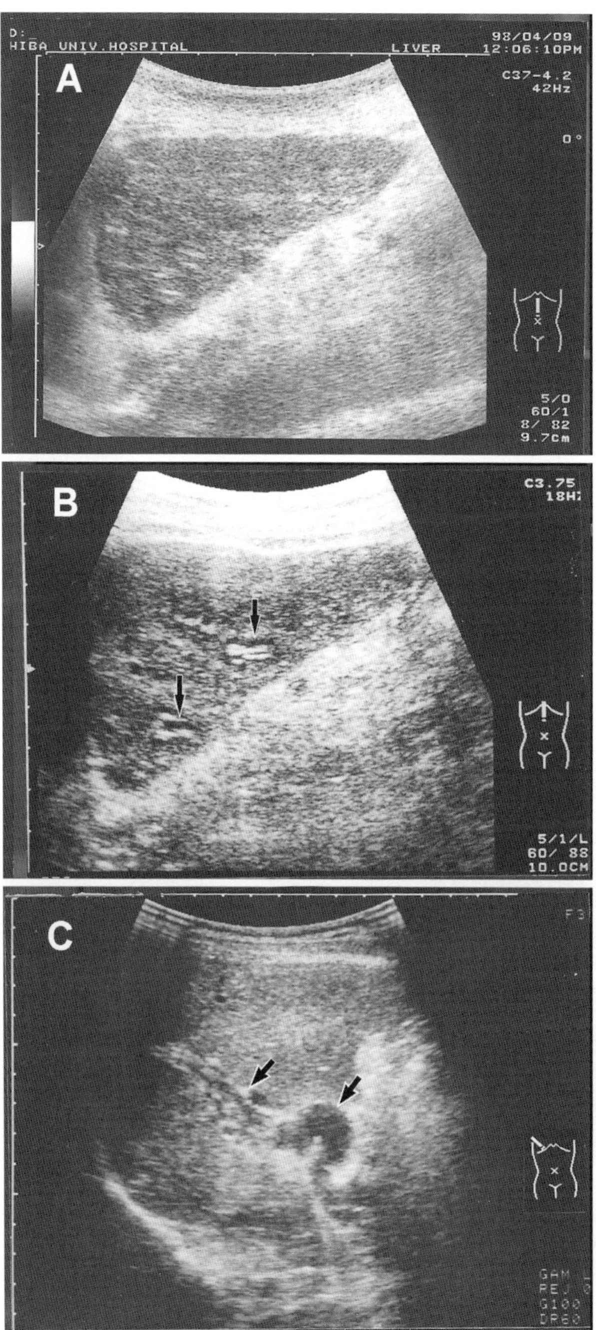

Fig. 5. Ultrasonograms of the diseases causing portal hypertension. For explanation, see page 48.

References

1. Lebrec D. Methods to evaluate portal hypertension. Gastroenterol Clin North Am 1992;21: 41–59.
2. Bolondi L, Piscaglia F, Siringo S, Giani S, Zironi G. Imaging techniques and hemodynamic measurement in portal hypertension. In: Franchis RD (ed) Portal Hypertension II. Oxford: Black-well Science, 1996;56–66.
3. Komaiko MS. Spleen imaging. In: Hiatt JR, Phillips EH, Morgenstern L (eds) Surgical Disease of the Spleen. Berlin: Springer-Verlag, 1997;61–87.
4. Matsutani S, Kimura K, Ohto M, Okuda K. Ultrasonography in the diagnosis of portal hypertension. In: Okuda K, Benhamou JP (eds) Portal Hypertension Clinical and Physiological Aspects. Tokyo: Springer-Verlag, 1991;197–206.
5. Okuda K, Takayasu K, Matsutani S. Angiography in portal hypertension. Gastroenterol Clin North Am 1992;21:61–83.
6. Matsutani S, Furuse J, Ishii H, Mizumoto H, Kimura K, Ohto M. Hemodynamics of the left gastric vein in portal hypertension. Gastroenterology 1993;105:513–518.
7. Matsutani S, Mizumoto H, Fukuzawa T, Ohto M, Okuda K. Response of blood flow to vasopressin in the collateral left gastric vein in patients with portal hypertension. J Hepatol 1995; 23:557–562.
8. Bude RO, Rubin JM. Power Doppler sonography. Radiology 1996;200:21–23.
9. Ferrara K, DeAngelis G. Color flow mapping. Ultrasound Med Biol 1997;23:321–345.
10. Matsutani S, Maruyama H, Ebara M, Yoshikawa M, Saisho H, Ohto M. Contrast-enhanced color Doppler in the diagnosis of liver tumors. In: Nanda NC, Schlief R, Goldberg BB (eds) Advances in echo imaging using contrast enhancement. Dordrecht: Dordrecht Kluwer Academic Publishers, 1997;627–634.
11. Dilton EH, van Leeuwen MS, Fernandes A, Mali WPTM. Spiral CT angiogaphy. AJR 1993; 160:1273–1278.
12. Zeman RK, Silverman PM, Vieco PT, Costello P. CT angiography. AJR 1995;165:1079–1088.
13. Edelman RR, Zhao B, Liu C, Wentz KU, Mattle HP, Fin JP, McArdle C. MR angiography and dynamic flow evaluation of the portal venous system. AJR 1989;153:755–760.

Progress in Hepatology, Volume 4.
Liver Cirrhosis Update.
M. Yamanaka et al., editors.

51

Endoscopic treatment for esophagogastric varices

H. Suzuki, M. Yamamoto, K. Hachiya and S. Hino
Department of Endoscopy, Jikei University School of Medicine, Tokyo, Japan

Abstract. This paper is focused on the endoscopic strategy for esophageal varices. In 1980, endoscopic injection sclerotherapy (EIS) with the use of a flexible fiberscope was introduced as a strategy of dealing with this particular disease.

EIS has been a standard procedure for more than 15 years, however, the technique itself is sometimes not so easy and more than a few systemic complications may arise, such as perforation, sepsis, pneumonia, portal emboli, and so forth. To prevent these complications, endoscopic variceal ligation (EVL) was introduced. Recently, combined therapy with EIS and EVL has become a standard strategy. Color Doppler endoscopic ultrasonography (CD-EUS) is very helpful in detecting the effect of endoscopic or radiologic interventional treatments. Furthermore, we are developing a new strategy, ICG-enhanced diode laser (805-nm wave length) therapy for the complete eradication of varices.

Keywords: color Doppler endoscopic ultrasonography (CD-EUS), endoscopic injection sclerotherapy (EIS), endoscopic variceal ligation (EVL), histoacryl, pneumoactive EVL device.

Introduction

Recently, endoscopic injection sclerotherapy (EIS) for esophageal varices with the use of a flexible endoscope was evaluated as the first-line therapeutic modality. However, there are many sclerosants and injection techniques and we have not found any standard technique yet. In Europe and Japan, 5% ethanolamine oleate and 1% polidocanol are commonly used, while sodium morrhuate and sodium tetradecyl are generally employed in the USA. The indications for the use of the treatment, especially for prophylactic therapy, are still controversial. In Japan, prophylactic sclerotherapy is commonly applied to nonbleeders if they have endoscopic risky varices. The Japanese Society for Portal Hypertension and Esophageal Varices published the general rules for recording endoscopic findings on esophageal varices initially in 1980 [1] and then in 1992 [2] as the revised edition. The rules consist of six main categories such as location (L), form (F), color (C), red color (RC) sign, bleeding sign and mucosal findings. All esophagogastric (EG) varices observed by endoscopy are recorded with this latest classification to enable easy discussion and evaluation of the patient's status and therapeutic results among the difference endoscopists and/or institutions. A statistical study showed us that the risky signs to look for are varices larger than F_2, associated with red color signs; and a prospective randomized multicenter trial

---

Address for correspondence: H. Suzuki MD, Department of Endoscopy, Jikei University School of Medicine, 25-8, 3 Chome, Nishi-Shinbashi, Minato-ku, Tokyo 105-8461, Japan.

52

regarding the efficacy of EIS is ongoing in Japan. However, most other countries doubt its efficacy, since 70% of variceal patients will not have variceal bleeding during their lifetime.

Seventeen years experience of our sclerotherapies with the combined para- and intravariceal injection technique using 1% polidocanol (Aethoxysklerol) [3], confirmed more than 90% efficacy of both hemostasis and eradication of varices. However, we thereafter introduced new endoscopic variceal treatments including polymer injection, endoscopic variceal ligation (EVL) and the combination of endoscopic ligation and sclerotherapy [4] to seek more effective and safer technique. This paper will be focused on the techniques and the results of our EIS, EVL and their combination therapy.

EIS using 1% polidocanol

From March 1979 to December 1990, we performed EIS on a total of 477 patients [3]. There were 149 emergent, 126 elective and 202 prophylactic cases and in terms of the child's classification, 98 patients were classified as child A, 205 were classified as child B and 174 were classified as child C. We chose 1% polidocanol as a sclerosant since it is easy and safe to inject, and our original para- and intravariceal injection technique. A freehand method, a technique without any balloon, overtube or sheath, was employed to simplify the procedure.

Sclerotherapy is performed under intravenous conscious sedation with diazepam or flunitrazepam and topical hypopharyngeal anesthetics (xlylocaine). A complete examination of the esophagus, stomach and duodenum was performed in all patients to detect esophageal varices and to exclude other nonvariceal bleeding. Then a 23 or 25 gauge fine injector needle filled with the sclerosant was inserted through the endoscopic working channel. Polidocanol is initially injected into the subepithelial layer of the esophagus between each varix slightly cephalad to the EG junction, and this is followed by an injection about 5 cm oral to the EG junction in the same fashion (Fig. 1). This procedure decreases variceal blood flow as well as replacing the esophageal wall with fibrotic tissue (sclerosis). Polidocanol is then injected directly into the varices and at this moment, the back flow of blood to the injector needle is observed. The dose of sclerosant for each injection is 3 ml and the total dose should be limited to 30 ml in each sclerotherapy to prevent local and systemic complications such as esophageal perforation, mediastinitis, hemolysis and so forth. Usually, three or four therapies were required to obtain complete eradication. Follow-up endoscopy is recommended every 3—6 months for early detection of variceal recurrence. Additional sclerotherapy is considered if the RC sign appears.

A common eradication course after sclerotherapy is as follows (Fig. 1):
1) shallow ulcers are formed on and around the injection site;
2) variceal channels are obliterated and varices are eradicated;
3) and fibrotic change (re-epithelialization) of the esophageal wall is observed after a series of sclerotherapy.

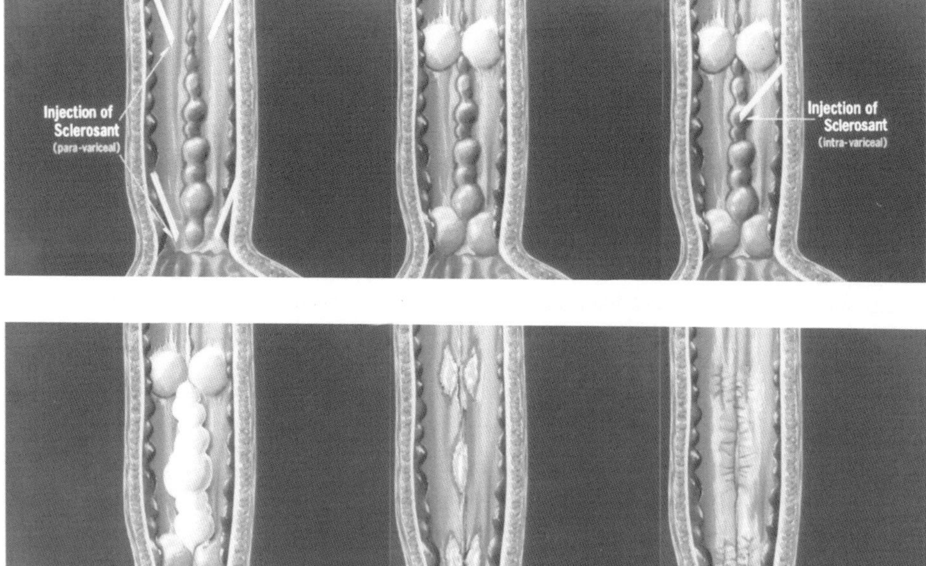

Fig. 1. The technique of endoscopic injection sclerotherapy, para- and intra-variceal injection technique. Common eradication course is demonstrated on the lower part. Courtesy of Jikei University.

Results of EIS

Of the 149 emergent patients, 93 had active bleeding at the emergent endoscopy and the bleeding was initially controlled in 86 patients resulting in a hemostatic rate of 92%. Even in patients with spurting bleeding, we obtained a hemostatic rate as high as 88%. On the other hand, out of 47 deaths, 17 patients (38%) died due to uncontrollable bleeding within a month.

Sclerotherapy is also performed to obtain complete eradication of the varices. Eradication was observed by endoscopy in 206 out of 229 patients followed up for more than 6 months and the efficacy rate was 90%. From the viewpoint of the variceal forms after sclerotherapy, rebleeding rates were significantly different. Among 23 patients who could not obtain satisfactory eradication (F_3 and F_2), the rebleeding rate was as high as 39.1% while in effective cases 12.2% (F_1) and 1.3% (F_0) rebled. From these results, the endpoint of sclerotherapy is the complete eradication (F_0) of varices. Rebleeding occurred in 55 patients out of 477 during the follow-up period. Forty-two patients rebled from the esophageal varices while 11 gastric varices were found as a bleeding source. Two patients bled from portal hypertensive gastropathy.

The long-term survival was evaluated by the Kaplan-Meier analysis. From the viewpoint of the therapeutic timing, survivals longer than 7.5 years were obtained in 54.6% of prophylactic, 39.2% of elective and 31.3% of emergent patients. Among the emergent cases, 74.3% of the child A group and 49.4% of the child B group survived for longer than 7.5 years while barely 18% of the child C group survived.

Local complications were experienced in 12 patients. There were six patients with esophageal strictures which were treated by single or multiple endoscopic balloon dilatation, one esophageal perforation treated conservatively and five patients with massive bleeding from postsclerosing ulcers. All ulcer bleedings, except one, were controlled by the heat probe, pure ethanol injection or additional sclerotherapy. There was no fatal systemic complications in our series.

EVL

EVL was developed by Stiegmann et al. [5] and is performed using a device which allows aspiration and ligation of varices using rubber bands (O rings). The advantage of this mechanical therapy is that there is no need for the injection of sclerosants or tissue glues and that it is able to avoid various complications known to be associated with injection therapies. EVL was introduced in Japan by the authors in 1989 [6] and 150 patients with esophageal varices and 20 with gastric varices had been treated by March 1995 [7].

In our initial experience of EVL, 20 out of 23 patients with esophageal varices showed an eradication effect as high as 87%. However, our aim for the therapy which is to achieve complete eradication (F0), could be observed only in five patients (21.7%).

At the present, our first-line procedure for the treatment of esophageal varices is called combined EVL-EIS therapy [8], that is, EVL with EIS using 1% polidocanol in the same series of treatment. However, EVL without sclerotherapy is still performed for patients with severe complications such as hepatic failure, renal failure, DIC and so forth.

Combined EVL-EIS therapy is performed in a manner similar to conventional sclerotherapy in sedated patients. An overtube, that allows repeated endoscopic insertion and withdrawals, is attached to the endoscope before the survey endoscopic examination. After the survey examination of the upper GI tract, the overtube is gently inserted, followed by the withdrawal of the endoscope. The EVL device is then mounted and the loaded endoscope is reinserted through the overtube.

Results of combined therapy

The overall outcome of the 150 patients treated by EVL-EIS therapy showed an eradication effect as high as 96%. From the viewpoint of the variceal form, there were 66 patients with F_3, 79 with F_2 and five patients had F_1 varices before the treatment. After a series of EVL-EIS therapy, these forms were improved to 6 patients with F_2, 67 with F_1 and 77 with F_0.

The details of the EVL-EIS therapy are as follows. EVLs were done over 180 sessions with an average of 1.2 sessions for each patient, and 1,530 ligations were attempted with 10.2 ligations per patient. Additional sclerotherapy was performed a total of 285 times and the average per patient was 1.9 sessions. Altogether, 3,800 ml of 1% polidocanol was injected and 25.3 ml was the average dose for the EVL-EIS therapy. This means that the injected sclerosant was decreased to a quarter of that used in sclerotherapy alone. For the 17 patients who had active bleeding at initial treatment, 100% hemostasis was obtained.

There were five complications that required endoscopic treatment, two esophageal strictures (1.3%) and three posttherapy bleedings (2.0%). Strictures were easily treated by single or multiple endoscopic dilatation and the bleedings were well-controlled by additional sclerotherapy. There were no deaths related to EVL-EIS therapy.

Recurrence of the varices was noted in 25 out of 41 patients (61%) who were followed up for more than 3 years. For such patients, additional endoscopic therapies were carried out mostly on an outpatient basis when recurrence was found. One or two sessions of low volume sclerotherapy are required to obtain satisfactory results without any complications.

A new pneumatic EVL device

EVL is very effective and easy to perform. However, we thought the original device needed a little modification to maximize the concept of the therapy. The list of the problems with the conventional device are as follows:
1) the visual field of the device attached to the endoscope is too narrow to observe the target varices and surroundings carefully;
2) the suction and/or irrigation to maintain a clear view during the treatment is limited since a trip wire occupies the endoscopic working channel;
3) and the ring is not always released when ligation is performed in a retroflexed fashion.

To solve these problems, we first made a transparent ligator with the cooperation of the original device manufactures. This modification was fairly effective and the visual field of the endoscope became 70% more than the gray-colored device. Then we also developed a new pneumatic EVL device consisting of a clear two-layer cylinder (an inner cylinder over which the O ring is stretched, and a sliding cylinder), an air tube and O ring plate [8]. This device pushes the O ring off with the sliding cylinder, which is activated by air injection, while the conventional device pulls a trip wire to move an inner cylinder toward the endoscope to release the ring. To load the device, the cylinder is first secured to the distal end of an endoscope followed by a thin air tube which connects the cylinder and an air injecting syringe, which is taped over the endoscope. This allows us to keep the endoscopic working channel clear with suction and irrigation or to insert an injector needle for simultaneous sclerotherapy. By this mechanism, the O ring can always be released even if the endoscope is fully retroflexed (Fig. 2).

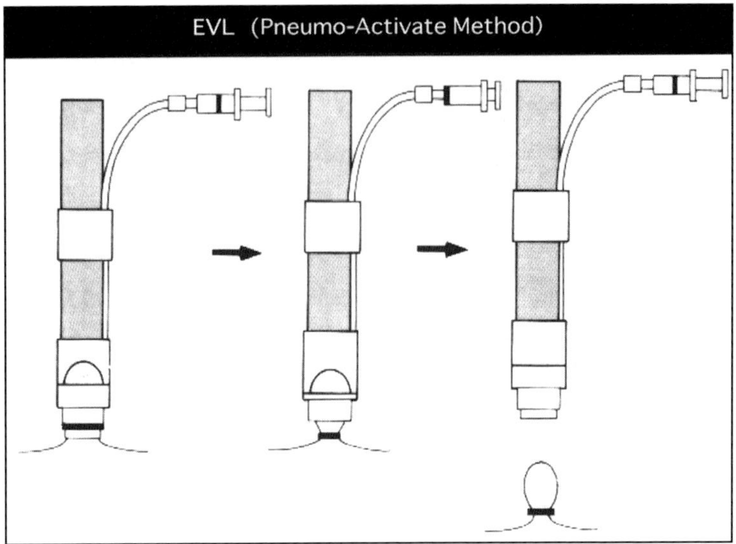

Fig. 2. Schema of EVL with the use of our original pneumoactive EVL device.

Moreover, the O ring plate of the pneumatic EVL device avoids complicated cylinder changing work and obviates the unexpected transmission of blood infectious diseases to medical personnel. The O ring plate has eight rubber bands and there is a preloading hole in the center of the plate to load and reload the O ring smoothly. Prior to each O ring loading, the device should be inserted to the preloading hole to push the sliding cylinder back to the working position. Then move the device onto the O ring cylinder and push down vertically to complete the loading. From a questionnaire that we issued, it would appear that medical personnel appreciated this improvement very much more than we thought.

Insertion of an endoscopic overtube at the outset of the procedure facilitates withdrawal and reinsertion of the endoscope for multiple ligations and prevents unexpected aspiration of blood to the respiratory organs. However, complications related to the overtube insertion, such as esophageal injury or perforations, have been reported. To make EVL, we also developed a new flexible overtube which is made of thinner silicon than the original one and reinforced by spiral wire like the esophageal prosthesis. The tip of a flexible tube is cut obliquely to prevent esophageal injury, and at the proximal end antideflate film is placed to maintain a better visual field during EVL. Unfortunately, the pneumatic EVL device and the flexible overtube are currently only available in Japan due to a patent problem, but we expect that similar modifications will be done in each country so that safer and easier EVL can be performed for patients suffering from variceal bleeding.

EIS using histoacryl

Histoacryl (n-butyl-2-cyanoacrylate) is a tissue adhesive which immediately polymerizes on contact with blood. The clinical efficacy of histoacryl for bleeding varices was first reported by Soehendra et al. [9] who introduced sclerotherapy using histoacyrl in 1988.

Results

We treated a total of 55 actively bleeding patients by sclerotherapy using histoacryl [10]. There were three patients with early recurrent bleeding from esophageal varices and 52 bleeding from gastric varices. A hemostatic effect was immediately obtained in 100% of the patients with 0.5—1.5 ml injections of histoacryl. No bleeding deaths were experienced after this therapy was introduced. From our repeated endoscopic observations, the polymer of the injected histoacryl was excreted to the esophageal or gastric cavity as a foreign body within 7—12 weeks. There were no complications related to the histoacryl injection, including rebleeding during the polymer excretion period.

Discussion

EIS was first reported by Crafoord et al. [11] in 1939. Recently it has been widely accepted by clinicians after using fiberscope since nearly 1979. Sclerotherapy was accomplished by injecting sclerosant directly into the venous channel (intravariceal), beside the channel (paravariceal) or a combination of both. Our technique uses 1% polidocanol and is a combined injection technique. On the other hand, Takase et al. [12] uses 5% Ethanolamine oleate that is injected intravarically under fluoscopic control. Both of the techniques mentioned above are standard in Japan since the two sclerosants can be used in our health care system.

The effects of EVL have been examined experimentally using the Jensen's portal hypertensive canine model by Stiegmann et al. [13]. At 3 to 7 days following ligation of varices, slough of variceal tissue and shallow ulcerations were observed at all treatment sites. At 14 to 21 days after the treatment, there were minimal residual varices and no evidence of full-thickness esophageal injury. Sites where previously shallow ulcers had appeared were healed and microscopic findings showed full-thickness replacement of vascular structures in the submucosa with maturing scar tissue. An intense inflammatory response was present and re-epithelialisation of treated sites had occurred by 21 days. These authors felt that the shallow ulcers produced at each ligated site resulted in little risk of bleeding and probably represented evidence of an effective treatment.

EVL has been examined in both uncontrolled and prospective randomized studies comparing ligation with sclerotherapy. Goff et al. [14] studied 146 consecutive nonselected patients who had variceal hemorrhage who were treated with EVL for control of acute hemorrhage and were then serially treated to achieve

58

variceal eradication. The control of active variceal hemorrhage was accomplished in 94% of 33 patients who were actively bleeding at index endoscopy. Variceal obliteration was achieved in 79% of the 125 patients who remained in the trial for more than 30 days with a mean of 5.5 endoscopic treatment sessions. Recurrent hemorrhage occurred in 44% and the overall survival rate in the 146 patients who entered the study was 73% at mean follow-up of 1.5 months. A total of four treatment-related nonbleeding complications were observed. Data from prospective randomized trials support that EVL is at least as effective as sclerotherapy for prevention of recurrent hemorrhage and results in comparable survival while inflicting a minimum risk of nonbleeding complications.

Reveille et al. [15] combined EVL with low volume sclerotherapy and reported that combination therapy may theoretically result in more rapid variceal obliteration because of the additional effects of mechanical stasis (ligation) and intimal damage (sclerotherapy). Their experiment consisted of 46 patients and eradication was accomplished in 76% of the patients, with a mean of 3.1 treatment sessions. The rebleeding rate was 30% with one death resulting from hemorrhage. Overall survival during the short follow-up period was 85%. These results support the theory that more rapid eradication may be possible with combined ligation and low volume sclerotherapy. From our experiences, we consider that combination therapy is superior to EVL alone.

Endoscopic injection of histoacryl or isobutyl cyanoacrylate (Bucrylate) for the treatment of esophagi and gastric fundal varices was described by several European groups. These two agents are tissue adhesive which polymerize rapidly in the blood. The aim of polymer injection treatment is to effect more rapid control of active bleeding.

Soehendra et al. [9] reported the clinical use of histoacryl in 27 patients with actively bleeding esophageal varices, and in four with bleeding fundal varices. Early rebleed occurred 7 times in four patients and all the rebleeding episodes were controlled with repeat injection of histoacryl. Overall survival from the index hospitalization in 40 actively bleeding patients treated with histoacryl and/or polidocanol was as high as 82.5%. An additional 30 patients with fundal varices were treated electively with histoacryl injections. Their report concluded that one or two treatment sessions resulted in elimination of such varices without any complications.

Ramond et al. [16] reported 49 patients treated with Bucrylate injections and 15 patients were actively bled at the index treatment sessions. Hemorrhage was controlled in 14 patients and elective repeat injections were performed with Bucrylate at varying intervals. Rebleeding occurred in 37% of patients during the first 6 months of the follow-up and in 42% by 1 year. Survival at 6 months follow-up was 100% for child A, 63% for child B and 13% for child C patients. Survival for the entire group after 1 year was 53%.

Complications associated with tissue adhesive injection appear more severe than those observed with conventional sclerotherapy. The most alarming report is from See et al. [17] detailing two patients who developed strokes immediately following Bucrylate and contrast agent (Lipiodol) mixture injections. The neurological injury was shown by subsequent radiological studies to have resulted from dissemination of the tissue glue into the cerebral arterial system. Therefore, we consider that tissue-adhesive injections should not be performed with contrast agent mixture to prevent the possible dissemination of the polymer.

Based on our original data and the other data currently available, it would appear that polymer injection is very effective for control of acute variceal hemorrhage from either esophageal or gastric varices. However, its safety remains to be established and requires strict patient selection criteria. We limited the use of histoacryl to early recurrent bleeding from the esophageal varices and treated

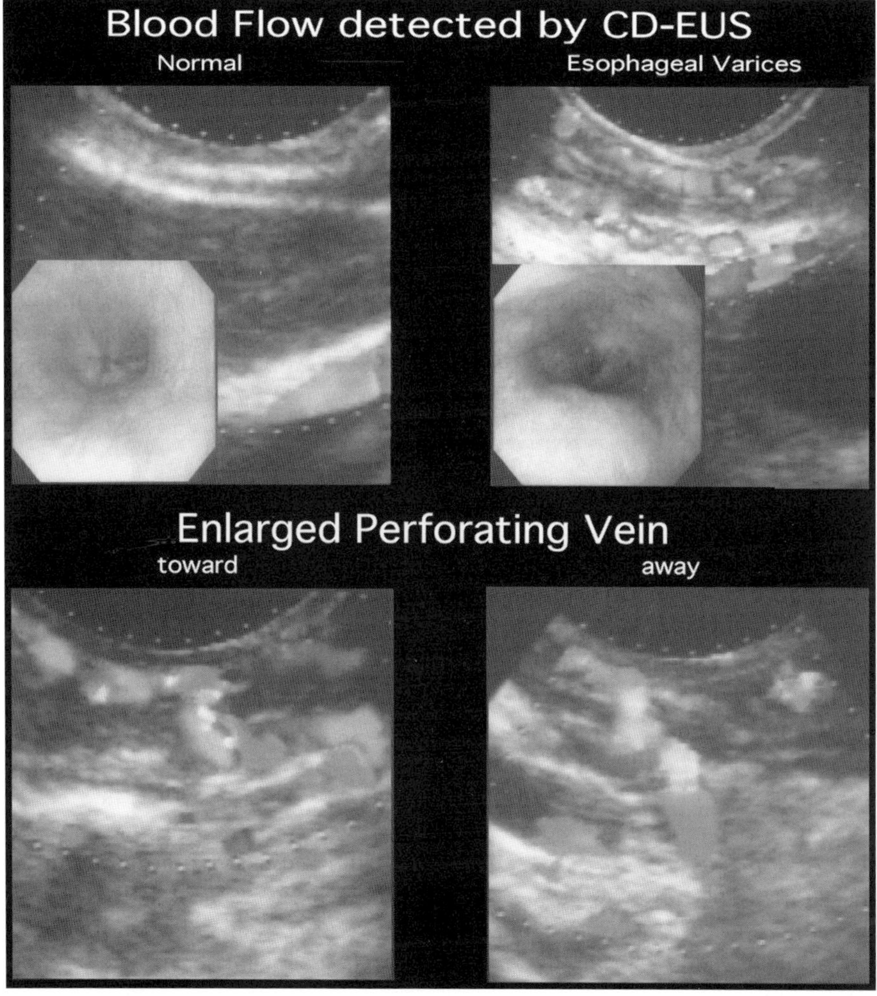

Fig. 3. Perforating vessels and intramucosal and paraesophageal veins can be detected by the CD-EUS.

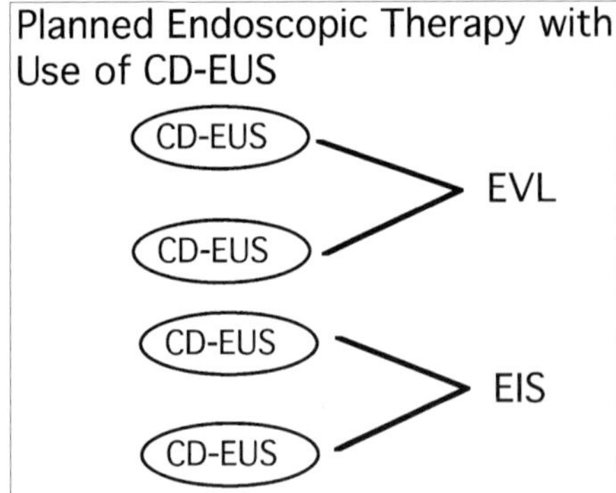

Fig. 4. Stepwise strategy in the treatment of esophageal varices using CD-EUS.

uncontrollable bleeding from gastric varices by conventional sclerotherapy.

Endoscopic treatment for esophageal varices is already an accomplished procedure but we should be trying to improve the technique and/or develop a new procedure to obtain better results. Recently, we introduced the color doppler endoscopic ultrasonography (CD-EUS) technique to detect the blood flow of varices and the important, perforating vessel (Fig. 3) and we are trying to perform the planned endoscopic therapy of esophageal varices with the use of CD-EUS (Fig. 4). Furthermore, we introduced a new laser treatment, namely, ICG enhanced Diode Laser Therapy to eradicate varices completely (Fig. 5). We con-

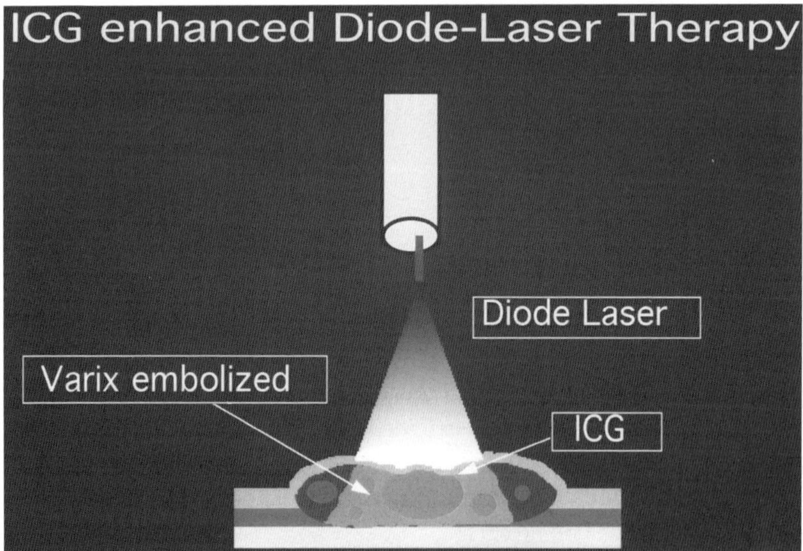

Fig. 5. ICG enhanced diode laser therapy was developed by the authors for the complete eradication of esophageal varices.

sider that the most important issue for the management of esophageal varices is having as many therapeutic options as possible and selecting the best therapy for each patient.

References

1. Japanese Research Society for Portal Hypertension. The general rule for recording endoscopic findings on esophageal varices. Jpn J Surg 1980;10:84—87.
2. Japanese Research Society for Portal Hypertension. The general rules for recording endoscopic findings on esophagogastric varices. Kanzou 1991;33:278. (In Japanese.)
3. Suzuki H, Yamamoto M. Endoskopische Sklerosierung und Varizenligatur zur Behandlung von Ocsophagus- und Magen Fundunvarizen. Chir Gastroenterol 1992;8:292—299.
4. Ohnishi T, Yamamoto M, Aoki T et al. Combination of endoscopic variceal ligation and endoscopic sclerotherapy with 1% polidocanol effect on esophageal varices. Prog Dig Endoscopy 1991;39:157—160. (In Japanese.)
5. Stiegmann GV, Sun JH, Hammond WS et al. A new endoscopic elastic band ligation device. Gastrointest Endosc 1986;32:230.
6. Yamamoto M, Suzuki H, Aoki T et al. Endoscopic variceal ligation. Endosc Dig 1990;2: 269—275. (In Japanese.)
7. Stiegmann GV, Yamamoto M. Endoscopic techniques for the management of active variceal bleeding. Gastrointest Endosc Clin North Am 1992;2:59—75.
8. Yamamoto M, Chibai M, Suzuki H. Esophageal and Gastric Variced. Tokyo: Nihon Medical Center, 1996;170—175. (In Japanese.)
9. Soehendra N, Grimm H, Nam VC et al. N-Butyl-2-Cyanoacrylate, a supplement to endoscopic sclerotherapy. Endoscopy 1987;19:83—86.
10. Suzuki H, Yamamoto M, Chibai M et al. Sclerotherapy of gastric varices with Histoacryl. Prog Dig Endoscopy 1988;33:83—86. (In Japanese.)
11. Crafoord C, Frenckner P. New Surgical treatment of varicose vein of the esophagus. Acta Otolaryngol 1939;27:422—429.
12. Takase Y, Nakahara A. Endoscopic embolization of esophageal varices. Prog Dig Endoscopy 1978;13:34—37. (In Japanese.)
13. Stiegmann GV, Sun JH, Hammond WS. Results of experimental endoscopic esophageal variceal ligation. Am Surg 1988;54:105—108.
14. Gofl JS, Reveille RM, Stiegmann GV. Endoscopic sclerotherapy versus endoscopic variceal ligation, Esophageal Symptoms Complications and mobility. Am J Gastroenterol 1988;83: 1240—1244.
15. Reveille RM, Golf JS, Stiegmann GV et al. Combination of endoscopic variceal ligation (EVL) and low volume sclerotherapy (ES) for bleeding esophageal varices: A factor route to variceal eradication (abstract). Gastrointest Endosc 1991;37:243.
16. Ramond MJ, Valla D, Gotliel JP et al. Obturation endoscopique des varices oeso-gastrique le bucrylate. Gastroenterol Clin Biol 1986;10:575—579.
17. See A, Florent C, Lamy D et al. Accidents vascularts cerebraus apres obturation endoscopique des varices esophagienes par 1-isobutyl-2-cyanoacrylate ches deux malades. Gastroenterol Clin 1986;10:604—607.

Progress in Hepatology, Volume 4.
Liver Cirrhosis Update.
M. Yamanaka et al., editors.

63

Pathophysiology and treatment of cirrhotic ascites

Hiroshi Fukui, Masahito Uemura and Tadasu Tsujii

Third Department of Internal Medicine, Nara Medical University, Nara, Japan

Abstract. The pathogenesis of cirrhotic ascites is extremely complex, being associated with multiple factors which include hepatic, renal, systemic circulatory and neurohumoral factors. Increased renal salt and water retention, sinusoidal and portal hypertension, and hypoalbuminemia are the key events for ascites formation. Despite much controversy surrounding major hypotheses, the formation of ascites is considered to be a continuum involving both overflow and underfill mechanisms. Meticulous use of diuretics is important, because diuretics themselves may lead to relative vascular underfilling. The body oppression therapy, a maneuver to improve peripheral vasodilation and restore effective vascular volume, was proven to be useful for some patients with ascites. Although various therapeutic maneuvers for refractory ascites led to transient improvement of ascites, they did not essentially prolong survival of cirrhotics. Iatrogenic complications should be carefully avoided by assessing the merits and risks of treatment in individual patients.

Keywords: albumin, ascites, body oppression, diuretics, endotoxin, liver cirrhosis, paracentesis, transjugular intrahepatic portosystemic shunt, vascular underfilling.

Introduction

The pathogenetic events leading to ascites formation in patients with liver cirrhosis are extremely complex, being associated with multiple factors [1,2] which include hepatic venous outflow block, portal hypertension and hypoalbuminemia as hepatic factors, hyperdynamic circulation, peripheral vasodilation and decreased effective circulating blood volume as systemic circulatory factors, and enhanced salt and water reabsorption in proximal and distal nephron related to intrarenal haemodynamic derangement, and altered neurohumoral system as renal factors. A rational therapeutic approach to cirrhotic ascites should be based on an understanding of its pathogenesis.

Pathogenesis of ascites in cirrhosis

The underfilling theory and the overflow theory

Two main hypotheses have been proposed to explain the mechanism of ascites formation: the underfilling theory and the overflow theory. In the former, excess lymph accumulation in the peritoneal space such as ascites is considered to lead to contraction of circulating plasma volume, which is thought to constitute an

---

Address for correspondence: Hiroshi Fukui, Third Department of Internal Medicine, Nara Medical University, 840 Shiji-cho, Kashihara-shi, Nara 634, Japan.

afferent signal to the renal tubule to augment salt and water reabsorption [1]. In the latter, renal sodium retention and plasma volume expansion is considered to precede rather than follow the formation of ascites [3]. These two hypotheses have aroused much controversy. In addition, Schrier et al. [4] recently proposed the peripheral vasodilation theory as a revised underfilling theory. In this theory, peripheral vasodilation was considered to cause imbalance of capacitance and volume, which leads to diminished effective intravascular volume.

Renal disturbance

Renal vasoconstriction is a common finding in patients with cirrhosis and ascites and more intense in the renal cortex, which may lead to a reduction of renal blood flow and glomerular filtration rate (GFR) [5]. Free water clearance and urinary sodium excretion are markedly decreased in those with tense ascites. Water and sodium retention in advanced cirrhosis is due to increased tubular reabsorption. Increased reabsorption in the proximal tubule leads to a reduced delivery of filtrate. An additional increased reabsorption in the distal tubule may further enhance water and sodium retention.

Circulatory abnormalities

Cirrhotic patients exhibit the hyperdynamic circulation characterized by arterial hypotension, increased cardiac output, and reduced systemic vascular resistance [6]. These changes have been attributed to peripheral vasodilation and arterio-venous shunt. We have noted that creatinine clearance and urinary sodium excretion reduced as the peripheral vascular resistance decreased (unpublished data). The tendency to underfilling associated with peripheral vasodilation may induce compensatory responses such as mobilization of vasoactive hormones and activation of the sympathetic nervous system [7].

Role of neurohumoral systems

A wide variety of neurohumoral derangement may influence renal handling of salt and water [7]. The activities of the two major vasoconstrictor and anti-natriuretic systems, the renin-angiotensin-aldosterone system and the sympathetic nervous system, are increased in most cirrhotics with tense ascites [5]. Increased plasma level of antidiuretic hormone (ADH) enhances water reabsorption in the collecting duct and contributes to water retention [5]. Endothelin, an endothelial-derived peptide with marked vasoconstrictor activity, is also increased in advanced cirrhosis [8,9]. Increased endothelin levels were proven to be related to creatinine clearance, effective renal plasma flow [10], serum creatinine and blood pressure [11], and may contribute to renal dysfunction in patients with cirrhosis [10].

On the other hand, α-human atrial natriuretic peptide (α-hANP) is considered to be increased as a homeostatic mechanism to counteract the effects of anti-natriuretic and vasoconstrictor systems in the renal circulation [12]. However, at the advanced stage of disease, it is suggested that the kidney is relatively resistant to natriuretic action of ANP and that elevated levels of ANP are insufficient to counterbalance antinatriuretic forces [13]. Increased renal production of vasodilator prostaglandins (PGs), especially PGE2, contributes to the maintenance of renal hemodynamics in cirrhotic ascites [14]. Likewise, the renal kallikrein-kinin system may contribute to the homeostatic modulation of renal function [15]. Reduced urinary excretion of vasodilator PGE2 and increased urinary excretion of vasoconstrictor thromboxan B2 were reported in patients with ascites and hepatorenal syndrome [16]. A recent finding of considerable interest was that systemic and renal nitric oxide (NO) activity was elevated in patients with liver cirrhosis. However, the cirrhotic kidney seems to be refractory to the natriuretic effect of this potent vasodilator. Intrarenal increase in NO may also be a compensatory mechanism against the stimulation of antinatriuretic systems [17].

Treatment of ascites in cirrhosis

Diuretics

The rational basis of diuretic therapy lies in an understanding of mechanisms and sites of action of the diuretic agents [18]. Two types of natriuretic agents are commonly used for the treatment of ascites: 1) drugs that inhibit sodium transport in the ascending limb of the loop of Henle (loop diuretics); and 2) agents that block the sodium-retaining arm of the renin-angiotensin-aldosterone system (distal diuretics, aldosterone antagonists) [19]. A stepped care medical approach consisting of bed rest, low-sodium diet, and the administration of aldosterone antagonists and loop diuretics is widely accepted for the management of cirrhotic ascites [20—22]. Although most European authors [20,23,24] described that the recommended dosage of spironolactone and furosemide in the treatment of cirrhosis with ascites was 100—500 mg/day and 40—240 mg/day, respectively, we frequently experience electrolyte disturbance or azotemia in our Japanese patients by a single high-dose diuretic treatment. In order to avoid diuretic-induced side effects, we designed our stepped care protocol with a combination of low-dose aldosterone antagonists and loop diuretics on the basis of salt restriction [25].

Fifty-four patients with liver cirrhosis and ascites were enrolled and stepped care diuretic treatment was performed as follows: step 1, placed on a 35 mEq sodium diet; step 2, given 400 mg/day of potassium canrenoate in addition to step 1 treatment; step 3, given 40—80 mg/day of furosemide in addition to step 2 treatment. Each step was performed for at least 7 days. Patients who did not experience ascites mobilization or who showed poor response were placed on the next step of treatment. At step 3, the dosage of furosemide was increased to

80 mg/day when ascites were not decreased by the dose of 40 mg/day. Albumin was intravenously supplemented if serum albumin levels became < 3.0 g/dl. As a result, 11 out of 54 patients (20.3%, group 1), 21 patients (38.9%, group 2) and seven patients (13.0%, group 3) lost their ascites at steps 1, 2 and 3, respectively. The remaining 15 patients (27.8%) did not respond to step 3 treatment. In group 1 patients, basal renal function was almost normal (Fig. 1) and basal plasma renin activity (PRA), basal plasma levels of aldosterone (PAC), and norepinephrine (NE) were within normal limits (Fig. 2). Urinary sodium excretion (UNaV), which was normal when they had ascites, was decreased under sodium restriction. Excessive sodium intake seemed to be responsible for the develop-

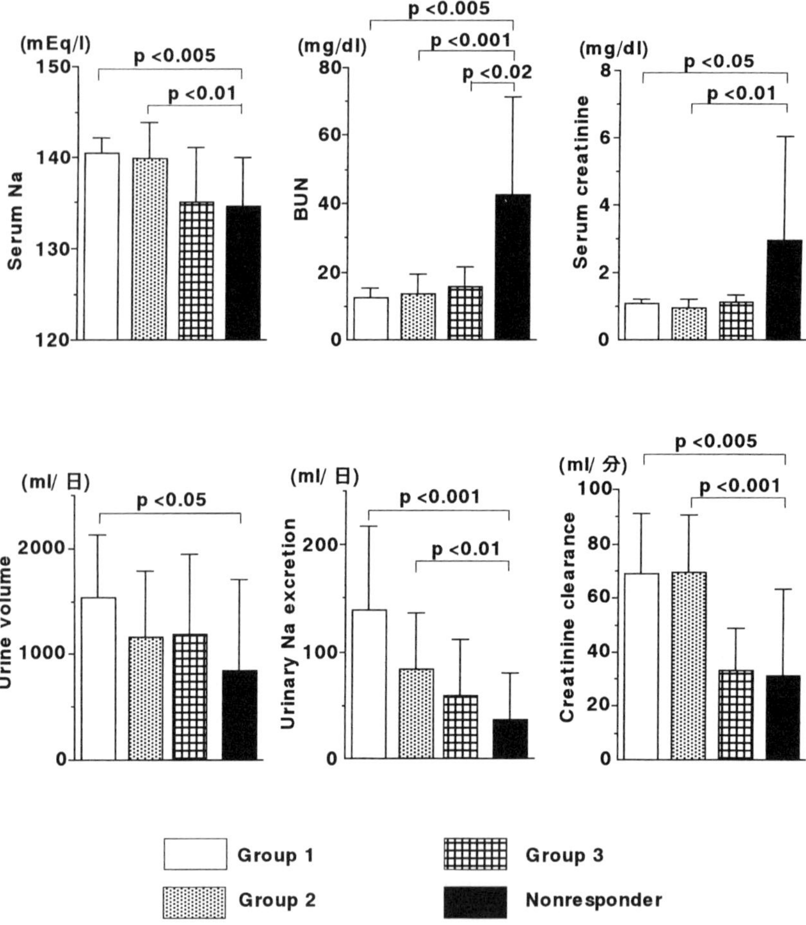

Fig. 1. Basal serum Na, BUN, serum creatinine, urine volume, urinary Na excretion and creatinine clearance in four groups of patients who received stepped care medical treatment of ascites. Group 1, group 2 and group 3 mean patients who lost ascites at step 1, step 2 and step 3, respectively.

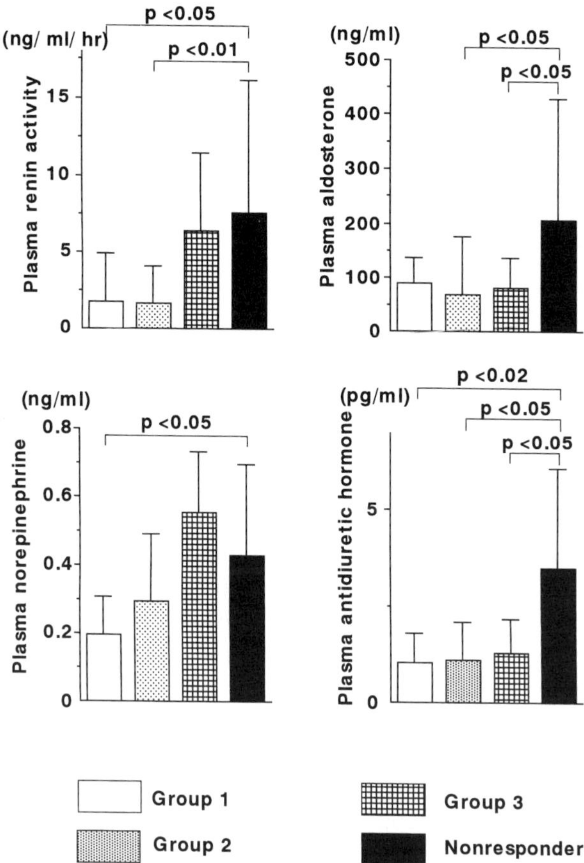

Fig. 2. Basal plasma renin activity, alsdosterone, norepinephrine and antidiuretic hormone in four groups of patients who received stepped care medical treatment of ascites. Group 1, group 2 and group 3 mean patients who lost ascites at step 1, step 2 and step 3, respectively.

ment of ascites in these patients, because they had been on a conventional Japanese diet that usually contained 15–25 g/day NaCl. In group 2 patients, basal plasma α-hANP level was elevated (Fig. 2), and basal PRA, PAC and NE in most of these patients were within normal range as in the group 1 patients (Fig. 2). The changes in hormonal parameters after step 2 treatment showed an increase in PRA, PAC and NE (Fig. 3) and a decrease in α-hANP levels (Fig. 4), suggesting that K canrenoate may lead to relative vascular underfilling in group 2 patients, who were initially in the overflow state. Group 3 patients showed decreased creatinine clearance (Ccr) and UNaV before the treatment (Fig. 1). Basal PRA and plasma NE were somewhat elevated in these patients (Fig. 2). Plasma α-hANP levels in group 3 patients were lower than those in group 2 (Fig. 2).

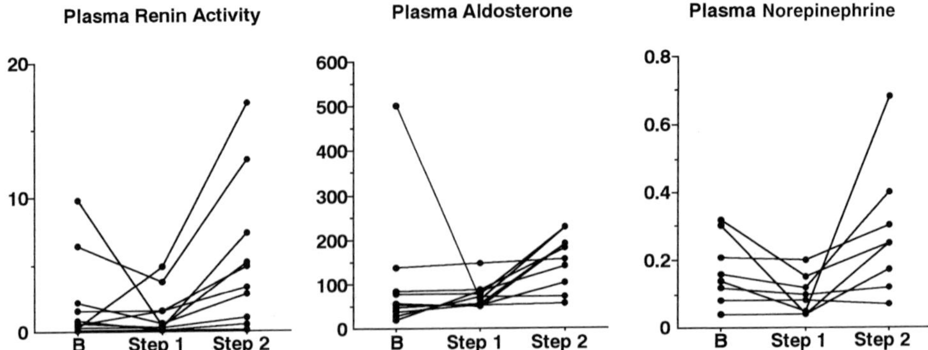

Fig. 3. Changes in plasma renin activity, plasma aldosterone concentration and plasma norepinephrine concentration before and after each step of treatment in group 2 patients [25]. B = before treatment; step 1, after step 1 treatment; step 2, after step 2 treatment.

In nonresponders, the decreases in serum Na, urine volume, UNaV and Ccr were remarkable (Fig. 1). In this group, increases in blood urea nitrogen, serum creatinine, PRA, PAC, NE and antidiuretic hormone (ADH) were significant (Figs. 1 and 2). These hormonal changes in group 3 patients and nonresponders were consistent with the state of vascular underfilling in the development of ascites.

The formation of ascites is considered to be a continuum involving both overflow (early, groups 1 and 2) and underfill (late, group 3 and nonresponder) mechanisms [25]. In this stepped care protocol, no patients developed electrolyte disturbance or diuretic-induced uremia, although serum K was slightly elevated

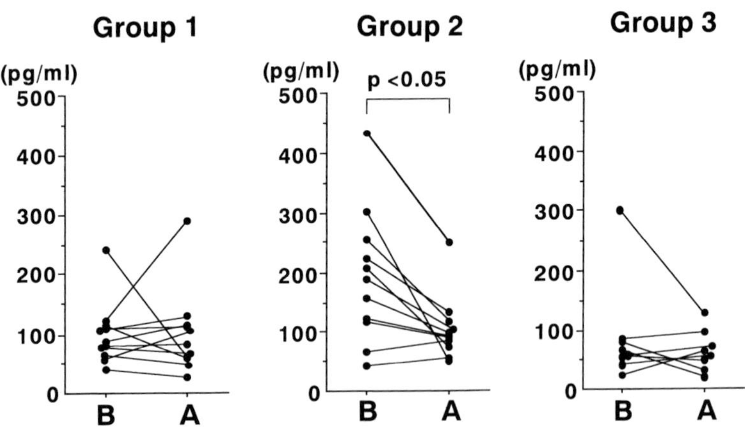

Fig. 4. Changes in plasma α-human atrial natriuretic polypeptide before and after stepped care treatment in three groups [25]. Group 1, group 2 and group 3 mean patients who lost ascites at step 1, step 2 and step 3, respectively. B = before treatment; A = after treatment.

after step 2 treatment [25]. In our preliminary study, patients who took more K canrenoate developed hyperkalaemia and decreased Ccr, indicating that 400 mg/day of K canrenoate could be regarded as the maximal antimineralocorticoid dosage to be reached before the addition of loop diuretics [25]. In addition, we first gave 40–80 mg furosemide to several cirrhotics with ascites who did not respond to salt restriction. The elevations of PRA and plasma NE noted then were more pronounced than those induced by 400 mg/day of K canrenoate, suggesting furosemide-induced rapid vascular underfilling. These data indicate that our stepped care medical treatment with 400 mg/day of K canrenoate and additional furosemide is a rational approach to cirrhotic patients with ascites. The responder to sodium restriction or potassium canrenoate was considered to be in the state of vascular overflow, while the nonresponders to K canrenoate were considered to be in the state of vascular underfilling. By the way, we have observed that diuretics themselves may lead to relative vascular underfilling.

From these observations, we considered that a maneuver to restore effective vascular volume may be necessary for patients with intractable ascites in the state of severe vascular underfilling.

Body oppression therapy

Epstein et al. [26] first reported the head-out water immersion (HWI) as a unique means to restore the reduced effective blood volume in cirrhotic patients. The HWI induced a prompt redistribution of circulating blood volume with a relative central hypervolemia and was associated with a profound and progressive natriuresis and diuresis with the suppression of the renin-angiotensin system in patients with liver cirrhosis and ascites [27]. However, the problem with the HWI is that patients need a big water bath and outpatients cannot easily receive this therapy. Thereafter, we applied the principle described by Epstein et al. [26,27] and designed a "body oppression" by using the stroke rehabilitation splints as an alternative means to restore the reduced effective blood volume in cirrhotic patients [28].

We have investigated the effect of "body oppression" on several parameters related to ascites formation in cirrhotics [28]. All patients were maintained on a constant sodium diet of 85 mEq per day for at least 7 days. All were given spironolactone 50–75 mg/day and furosemide 40–80 mg/day. Eight cirrhotics lost ascites by diuretics and the remaining eight cirrhotics had ascites despite the administration of diuretics. Cirrhotic patients and healthy subjects always ate lunch at noon, and thereafter were instructed to take a supine position for 1 h. After voiding and completely emptying their bladders, the subjects received the body oppression in the supine position for 3 h (2.00 pm–5.00 pm). Four limbs and the lower abdomen of supine patients were oppressed with the constant pressure, height (cm) divided by 13.6 mmHg, for 3 h using stroke rehabilitation splints (Svend Andersen, Co., Ltd., Denmark). On the day prior to the body oppression, control data without the body oppression was taken under the same conditions.

70

As a result, urine volume (UV), UNaV and Ccr were significantly greater in the body oppression periods than those in the control periods, both in cirrhotics with and without ascites. Fractional excretion of sodium was significantly increased only in cirrhotics with ascites (mean 0.36–0.79, $p < 0.05$). In healthy subjects, these parameters tended to be increased, but their differences did not reach statistical significance. The percent changes of UV and UNaV were significantly greater in cirrhotics with ascites than those in cirrhotics without ascites (UV: means 124 vs. 63%, $p < 0.05$; UNaV: 132 vs. 53%, $p < 0.05$, respectively). PRA, AII, PAC and NE were significantly decreased both in cirrhotics without and with ascites (PRA: mean 5.2–3.0 ng/ml/h, $p < 0.05$ vs. 10.1–6.0 ng/ml/h, $p < 0.005$; AII: 36–22 pg/ml, $p < 0.05$ vs. 47–26 pg/ml, $p < 0.05$; PAC: 91–47 pg/ml, $p < 0.05$ vs. 153–103 pg/ml, $p < 0.05$; NE: 520–348 pg/ml, $p < 0.05$ vs. 950–573 pg/ml, $p < 0.01$, respectively). ADH decreased in two cirrhotics with high basal levels. In healthy subjects, these hormone levels tended to decrease. These data suggest that the improvement in renal function by the body oppression in cirrhotics is attributable to the central hypervolemia and the reversal of the elevated renal vascular tone in cirrhotics as noted in the HWI [26,27].

In addition, in order to estimate the effectiveness of the body oppression itself, six other cirrhotics with tense ascites and marked hypoalbuminemia (mean 2.4 g/dl) were treated with the body oppression for 3 h every day without any administration of diuretics or albumin. Three of them were responders whose ascites markedly improved with the gradual increase in UV and UNaV. The remaining three cirrhotics were nonresponders whose ascites did not ameliorate without any improvement in renal functions. The effectiveness of repeated body oppression for cirrhotic ascites depends on basal renal function of cirrhotics. In nonresponders, basal BUN was higher and basal UNaV and basal Ccr were lower as compared to those of responders (BUN: means 36 vs. 12 mg/dl, $p < 0.05$, UNaV: 8 vs. 30 mEq/day, $p < 0.05$, Ccr: 33 vs. 76 ml/min). These results suggested that the body oppression was not effective for those with severe renal disturbance.

With respect to the mechanism of central hypervolemia by the body oppression, the oppression of peripheral capillaries in four limbs and lower abdomen is considered to improve the arterial vasodilation and enhance shifts of the blood from the peripheral to the central area in cirrhotic patients.

Peritoneovenous shunt

LeVeen et al. [29] first introduced the peritoneovenous shunt for the treatment of ascites. The device allowed ascites infusion to the jugular vein by the one-way pressure-sensitive valve. The shunt has been demonstrated to be effective for patients with massive ascites, especially for those with relatively preserved hepatic function (serum total bilirubin less than 10 mg/dl, prothrombin time more than 40%) or for those without hepatic encephalopathy and gastrointestinal bleeding. Many observers have documented a marked diuresis together with an increase in renal blood flow and suppression of renin-angiotensin-aldosterone systems [30]. Interestingly, improved natriuresis by the shunt was accompanied by a return to diuretic responsiveness [30].

Despite these encouraging reports, there is a large number of serious complications such as disseminated intravascular coagulation, peritonitis, sepsis and cardiac failure.

Obstruction of the shunt was the most common problem during follow-up [31], which led to the introduction of a shunt with a pumping mechanism — the Denver shunt [30]. Zervos et al. [32] observed the long-term efficacy of Denver shunt and reported that the shunt provided palliation for intractable ascites in the short term, but commonly occluded within 1 year. They concluded that complications were high and survival was limited.

Ascites reinfusion

Reinfusion of filtered and concentrated ascites is safer than the conventional ascites reinfusion or peritoneovenous shunt. However, one problem related to this procedure is frequent endotoxemia attributable to concentrated endotoxin in ascites. We have noted that cirrhotic ascites contain a large amount of endotoxin, most of which are supposed to be bound and inactivated by ascites proteins. Decreased endotoxin-binding capacity of HDL and albumin in ascites are confirmed to be related to renal disturbance in cirrhotics.

Figure 5 shows plasma endotoxin concentration in a patient with refractory ascites. Although endotoxin in the filtered and concentrated ascites was absorbed

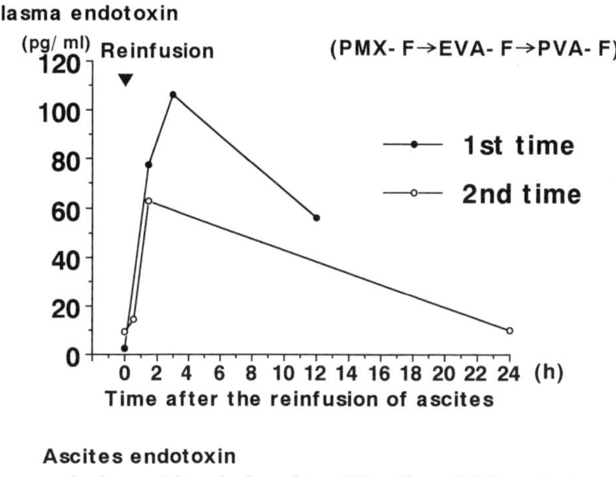

Fig. 5. Plasma endotoxin concentration after reinfusion of concentrated ascites in one patient with refractory ascites. Even polymixin-B column could not eliminate ascites endotoxin.

by polymixin-B column before reinfusion the resultant fluid still contained a high concentration of endotoxin, and plasma endotoxin level was elevated by the procedure. Serious complications associated with endotoxemia are very rare. However, the procedure should be contraindicated in patients with suspected spontaneous bacterial peritonitis. An alternative method is an intraperitoneal ascites reinfusion reported by Borzio et al. [33]. They reported that ascites concentration and reinfusion either intravenously or intraperitoneally did not adversely modify haemodynamic or renal parameters except for a transient decrease in mean arterial pressure, although a transient decrease in platelet count and serum fibrinogen levels and pyrexia were observed in patients reinfused intravenously.

Therapeutic paracentesis

Large volume-paracentesis was re-evaluated and the technique with intravenous albumin infusion was proved to be safe and useful for the cirrhotics with tense ascites [34,35]. Luca et al. [34] reported that in patients with cirrhosis and tense ascites total paracentesis favorably influences the systemic hemodynamics, portocollateral blood flow and portal pressure with a fall in the elevated levels of plasma renin activity, plasma aldosterone and plasma norepinephrine and a decrease in levels of serum creatinine and blood urea nitrogen. Kravetz et al. [36] noted the usefulness of total volume paracentesis in the treatment of variceal hemorrhage in that it produced a significant reduction in intravariceal pressure and variceal pressure gradient. The variceal size and variceal wall tension were also reduced. Pozzi et al. [37] observed a marked reduction of intra-abdominal, intrathoracic, right atrial, and pulmonary pressures after total paracentesis (250 ml/min) and albumin infusion (6 g/l ascites). Systemic vascular resistance and mean arterial pressure were slightly decreased by the procedure. Angueira et al. [35] reported an improvement in pulmonary function and symptoms after this procedure. However, Chang et al. [38] noted that diuretic treatment may be superior to large-volume paracentesis for those with nonalcoholic cirrhosis and tense ascites in terms of the oxygenation improvement as evaluated by $AaPO_2$. Nevertheless, the large volume-paracentesis may be associated with severe underfilling state and azotemia. It is advisable to stop or reduce diuretics by the procedure. Webster et al. [39] reported rare hemorrhagic complications probably due to the rupture of large intra-abdominal venous collateral associated with large-volume abdominal paracentesis.

In our study, the nonresponders to the large-volume abdominal paracentesis and albumin infusion showed higher Child-Pugh scores and lower plasma fibrinogen levels than the responder (Fig. 6). An episode of hepatic encephalopathy by the procedure was frequent only in the nonresponders (Fig. 6).

Transjugular intrahepatic portosystemic shunt (TIPS)

TIPS showed a dramatic effect for refractory ascites. However, the prognosis of

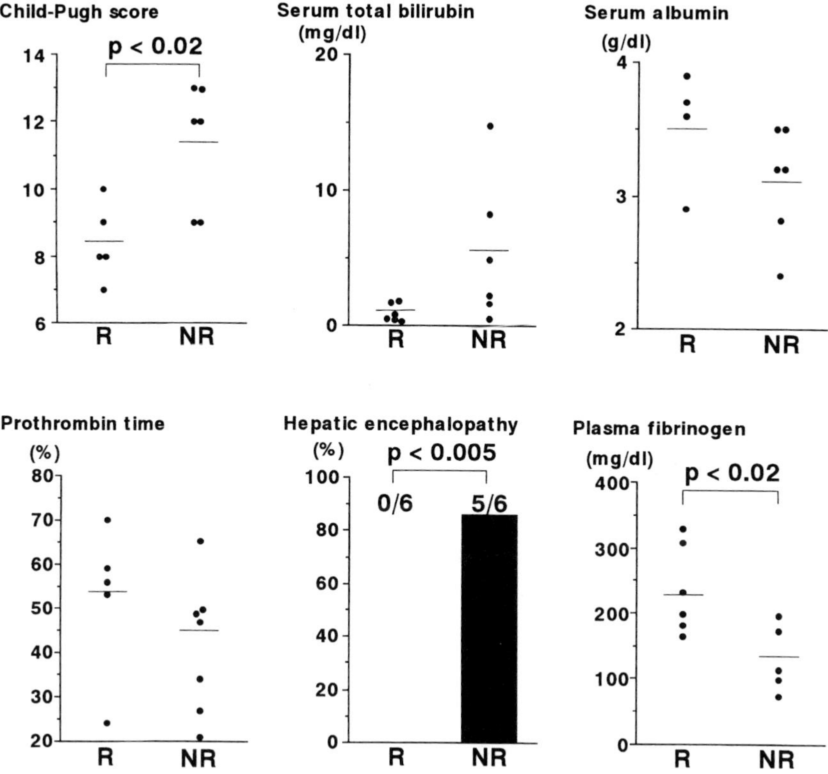

Fig. 6. Background factors which determine the responsiveness of ascites to the large volume abdominal paracentesis and albumin infusion. R = responder to the treatment; NR = nonresponder to the treatment; Hepatic encephalopathy: the incidence of hepatic encephalopathy during the treatment.

patients after the shunt was not necessarily satisfactorily associated with serious complications such as hepatic encephalopathy, deterioration of liver function or hepatic failure [20,21]. In the study of 17 patients by Quiroga et al. [40], five died and six received liver transplantation during the mean observation period of 15.6 months, although more than half of the ascites were improved, associated with an increase in natriuresis and suppression of renin, aldosterone and norepinephrine. Somberg et al. [41] selected five patients with tense ascites and mild hepatic and renal failure (serum total bilirubin lower than 5 mg/dl, serum creatinine lower than 2.5 mg/dl and platelet counts higher than 50,000 per mm^3). Marked improvement of ascites and renal function was observed, although one patient developed hepatic failure. In a large group of patients undergoing TIPS for refractory ascites by Ochs et al. [42], 46 of 50 were responders. However, two of the four nonresponders died within 2 weeks after the shunt. Survival for at least 1 year was associated with a patient being under 60 years of age; having a serum bilirubin level before placement of the stent shunt of less than 1.3 mg/dl. Wong et al. [43] suggested that old age and a parenchymal or functional renal dysfunction is associated with a lack of therapeutic response to TIPS.

Other reported complications of TIPS are transient intravascular hemolysis [44], deterioration of hyperdynamic state [45] and pulmonary hypertension [46]. Wong et al. [47] concluded that TIPS insertion should not be done in any patients with refractory ascites without paying careful attention to hepatic, cardiac, pulmonary and renal status, although they admitted that TIPS is a safe and effective means of managing refractory ascites. Nevertheless, careful consideration of hepatic reserve, underlying renal abnormalities, and cardiac and pulmonary function are necessary to assess the potential risks and benefits of TIPS [48].

Summary

Despite various new therapeutic approaches, ascites formation still remains a poor prognosis in patients with liver cirrhosis. Every trial to improve hepatic reserve capacity is mandatory for treatment of ascites in each patient. Iatrogenic complications should be carefully avoided by assessing the risks of treatment in individual patients.

References

1. Epstein M. Renal complications in liver disease. In: Schiff L, Schiff E (eds) Diseases of the Liver, 7th edn. Philadelphia: Lippincott, 1993;1016—1035.
2. Levy M. Pathophysiology of ascites formation. In: Epstein M (ed) The Kidney in Liver Disease, 3rd edn. Baltimore: Williams & Wilkins, 1988;209—243.
3. Liebermann F, Reynolds T. Plasma volume in cirrhosis of the liver: Its relation to portal hypertension, ascites and renal failure. J Clin Invest 1967;46:1297—1308.
4. Schrier RW, Arroyo V, Bernardi M et al. Peripheral arterial vasodilation hypothesis: A proposal for the initiation of renal sodium and water retention in cirrhosis. Hepatology 1988;8: 1151—1157.
5. Gines P, Fernandez-Esparrach G, Arroyo V et al. Pathogenesis of ascites in cirrhosis. Sem Liv Dis 1997;17:175—189.
6. Henriksen JH, Moller S. Hemodynamics, distribution of blood volume, and kinetics of vasoactive substances in cirrhosis. In: Epstein M (ed) The Kidney in Liver Disease, 4th edn. Philadelphia: Hanley & Belfus, Inc., 1996;241—258.
7. Levy M. Pathophysiology of ascites formation. In: Epstein M (ed) The Kidney in Liver Disease, 4th edn. Philadelphia: Hanley & Belfus, Inc., 1996;179—220.
8. Uchihara M, Izumi N, Sato C, Marumo F. Clinical significance of elevated plasma endothelin concentration in patients with cirrhosis. Hepatology 1992;16:95—99.
9. Asbert M, Gines A, Gines P et al. Circulating levels of endothelin in cirrhosis. Gastroenterology 1993;104:1485—491.
10. Tsai Y, Lin H, Yang M et al. Plasma endothelin levels in patients with cirrhosis and their relationships to the severity of cirrhosis and renal function. J Hepatology 1995;23:681—688.
11. Moller S, Emmeluth C, Henriksen JH. Elevated circulating plasma endothelin-1 concentrations in cirrhosis. J Hepatol 1993;19:285—290.
12. Fukui H, Tsujii T, Matsumura M et al. Plasma levels of atrial natriuretic peptide in patients with liver cirrhosis and its relation to ascites and renal function. Gastroenterol Jpn 1989;24:149—155.

13. Epstein M. Atrial natriuretic factor and liver disease. In: Epstein M (ed) The Kidney in Liver Disease, 4th edn. Philadelphia: Hanley & Belfus, Inc., 1996;339–358.
14. Uemura M, Tsujii T, Fukui H et al. Urinary prostaglandins and renal function in chronic liver diseases. Scand J Gastroenterol 1986;21:75–81.
15. Zipser RD, Radvan GH, Kronborg IJ et al. Urinary thromboxane B2 and prostaglandin E2 in the hepatorenal syndrome: Evidence of increased vasoconstrictor and decreased vasodilator factors. Gastroenterology 1983;84:697–703.
16. Perez-Ayuso RM, Arroyo V, Camps J et al. Renal kallikrein excretion in cirrhosis with ascites: relationship to renal hemodynamics. Hepatology 1984;4:247–252.
17. Romero JC, Garcia-Estan J, Atucha NM. Nitric oxide and renal function: the control of blood pressure under normal conditions and during cirrhosis. In: Epstein M (ed) The Kidney in Liver Disease, 4th edn. Philadelphia: Hanley & Belfus, Inc., 1996;373–385.
18. Epstein M. Diuretic therapy in liver disease. In: Epstein M (ed) The Kidney in Liver Disease, 4th edn. Philadelphia: Hanley & Belfus, Inc., 1996;447–458.
19. Bataller R, Arroyo V, Gines P. Management of ascites in cirrhosis. J Gastroenterol Hepatol 1997;12:723–733.
20. Epstein M. Diuretic therapy in liver disease. In: Epstein M (ed) The Kidney in Liver Disease, 3rd edn. Baltimore: Williams & Wilkins, 1988;537–550.
21. Arroyo V, Epstein M, Gallus G et al. Refractory ascites in cirrhosis: mechanism and treatment. Gasroenterol Int 1989;2:195–207.
22. Bernardi M, Laffi G, Salvagnini M et al. Efficacy and safety of the stepped care medical treatment of ascites in liver cirrhosis: a randomized controlled clinical trial comparing two diets with different sodium content. Liver 1993;13:156–162.
23. Angeli P, Caregaaro L, Menon F et al. Variability of atrial natriuretic peptide plasma levels in ascitic cirrhotics: Pathophysiological and clinical implications. Hepatology 1992;16:1389–1394.
24. Gatta A, Angeli P, Caregaro L, Menon F, Sacerdoti D, Merkel C. A pathophysiological interpretation of unresponsiveness to spironolactone in a stepped-care approach to the diuretic treatment of ascites in nonazotemic cirrhotic patients. Hepatology 1991;14:231–236.
25. Takaya A, Fukui H, Matsumura M et al. Stepped care medical treatment for cirrhotic ascites: analysis of factors influencing the response to treatment. J Gastroenterol Hepatol 1995;10:30–35.
26. Epstein M, Pins D, Schneider N et al. Determinants of deranged sodium and water homeostasis in decompensated liver cirrhosis. J Lab Clin Med 1976;87:822–839.
27. Epstein M. Renal sodium handling in liver diseases. In: Epstein M (ed) The Kidney in Liver Disease, 3rd edn. Baltimore: Williams & Wilkins, 1988;3–30.
28. Uemura M, Matsumoto M, Tsujii T et al. Effects of "body oppression" on parameters related to ascites formation and its therapeutic trial in cirrhotic patients. J Gastroenterology (In press).
29. Le Veen HH, Christoudias G, Moon JP et al. Peritoneovenous shunting for ascites. Ann Surg 1974;180:580–591.
30. Epstein M. Peritoneovenous shunt in the management of ascites and the hepatorenal syndrome. In: Epstein M (ed) The Kidney in Liver Disease, 4th edn. Philadelphia: Hanley & Belfus, Inc., 1996;491–506.
31. LeVeen HH, Vujic I, D'Ovidio NJ et al. Peritoneovenous shunt occlusion. Etiology, diagnosis, therapy. Ann Surg 1984;200:212–223.
32. Zervos EE, McCormick J, Goode SE et al. Peritoneovenous shunts in patients with intractable ascites: palliation at what price? Am Surg 1997;63:157–162.
33. Borzio M, Romagnoni M, Sorgato G et al. A simple method for ascites concentration and re-infusion. Dig Dis Sci 1995;40:1054–1059.
34. Luca A, Feu F, Garcia-Pagan J et al. Favorable effects of total paracentesis on splanchnic hemodynamics in cirrhotic patients with tense ascites. Hepatology 1994;20:30–33.
35. Angueira C, Kadakia S. Effects of large-volume paracenthesis on pulmonary function in

patients with tense ascites. Hepatology 1994;20:825–828.

36. Kravetz D, Romero G, Argonz J et al. Total volume paracentesis decreases variceal pressure, size, and variceal wall tension in cirrhotic patients. Hepatology 1997;25:59–62.

37. Pozzi M, Osculati G, Boari G et al. Time course of circulatory and humoral effects of rapid total paracentesis in cirrhotic patients with tense, refractory ascites. Gastroenterology 1994;106:709–719.

38. Chang S, Chang H, Chenl F et al. Therapeutic effects of diuretics and paracentesis on lung function in patients with non-alcoholic cirrhosis and tense ascites. J Hepatology 1997;26:833–838.

39. Webster ST, Brown KL, Lucey MR et al. Hemorrhagic complications of large volume abdominal paracentesis. Am J Gastroenterol 1996;91:366–368.

40. Quiroga J, Sangro B, Nunez M et al. Transjugular intrahepatic portosystemic shunt in the treatment of refractory ascites: Effect on clinical, renal, hormonal and hemodynamic parameters. Hepatology 1995;21:986–994.

41. Somberg K, Lake J, Tomlanovich S et al. Transjugular intrahepatic portosystemic shunts for refractory ascites: Assessment of clinical and hormonal response and renal function. Hepatology 1995;21:709–716.

42. Ochs A, Rossle M, Haag K et al. The transjugular intrahepatic portosystemic stent-shunt procedure for refractory ascites. N Engl J Med 1995;332:1192–1197.

43. Wong F, Sniderman K, Liu P, Blendis L. The mechanism of the initial natriuresis after transjugular intrahepatic portosystemic shunt. Gastroenterology 1997;112:899–907.

44. Sanyal AJ, Freedman AM, Purdum PP et al. The hematologic consequences of transjugular intrahepatic portosystemic shunts. Hepatology 1996;23:32–39.

45. Rodriguez LJ, Banares R, Echenagusia A et al. Effects of transjugular intrahepatic portasystemic shunt (TIPS) on splanchnic and systemic hemodynamics, and hepatic function in patients with portal hypertension. Preliminary results. Dig Dis Sci 1995;40:2121–2127.

46. Van der Linden P, Le Moine O, Ghvsels M et al. Pulmonary hypertension after transjugular intrahepatic portosystemic shunt: effects on right ventricular function. Hepatology 1996;23:982–987.

47. Wong F, Blendice L. Transjugular intrahepatic portosystemic shunt for refractory ascites: Tipping the sodium balance. Hepatology 1995;22:358–364.

48. Somberg KA. Transjugular intrahepatic portosystemic shunt in the treatment of refractory ascites and hepatorenal syndrome. In: Epstein M (ed) The Kidney in Liver Disease, 4th edn. Philadelphia: Hanley & Belfus, Inc., 1996;507–516.

Liver cirrhosis and disseminated intravascular coagulation

Kenji Fujiwara and Satoshi Mochida
Third Department of Internal Medicine, Saitama Medical School, Moroyama-cho, Iruma-gun, Saitama, Japan

Abstract. The hepatic sinusoid is a unique microvessel system in which endothelial cells express minimal tissue factor pathway inhibitor (TFPI) and thrombomodulin. Fibrin deposition in the hepatic sinusoids can cause massive liver necrosis. In cirrhotic liver, capillarized endothelial cells express increased thrombomodulin, but blood coagulation equilibrium can be easily deranged, because tissue factor activity is increased in hepatic macrophages after activation, while plasma antithrombin (AT) III activity is markedly decreased. Thus, disseminated intravascular coagulation (DIC) prevails on complication of bacterial infections in cirrhotic patients. Serial measurements of peripheral platelet count would be helpful for early diagnosis of DIC in cirrhotic patients. When peripheral platelet count is gradually decreased without any other cause, continuous infusion of synthetic protease inhibitors should be started. In the case of acute fulminant DIC, infusion of AT III concentrate is an essential therapy, but use of heparin or low-molecular-weight heparin is contraindication. Experimentally intravenous injection of recombinant human TFPI as well as oral administration of polymyxin B sulfate are therapeutic candidates for such DIC.

Keywords: antithrombin III, disseminated intravascular coagulation, sinusoidal endothelial cells, thrombomodulin, tissue factor, tissue factor pathway inhibitor.

Blood coagulation equilibrium in the hepatic sinusoids and its derangement

Blood coagulation cascade is triggered by tissue factor after its binding to activated blood coagulation factor VII (VIIa) resulting in activation of factor IX and X on phospholipid bilayers (Fig. 1) [1]. Tissue factor is expressed on monocytes, endothelial cells and tumor cells [1], suggesting that these cells can act thrombogenic in the microvessels. In normal conditions, the activation of blood coagulation cascade is suppressed by a variety of antithrombogenic factors expressed on endothelial cells (Fig. 2) [2]. Tissue factor pathway inhibitor (TFPI) plays a role in suppression of the upper stream of the cascade through inhibition of catalytic activity of factor VIIa and tissue factor complex on factor X and IX in a two-step feedback reaction with participation of activated factor X (Xa) and IXa (IXa) [3]. When the cascade is triggered by tissue factor increasing on monocytes and tumor cells, thrombomodulin immediately inactivates thrombin by forming a complex with thrombin which can activate protein C, and maintains antithrombogenic activity on endothelial cells [2].

Address for correspondence: Kenji Fujiwara MD PhD, Third Department of Internal Medicine, Saitama Medical School, 38 Moroyongo, Moroyama-cho, Iruma-gun, Saitama 350-0495, Japan. Tel.: +81-492-76-1198. Fax: +81-492-94-8404.

78

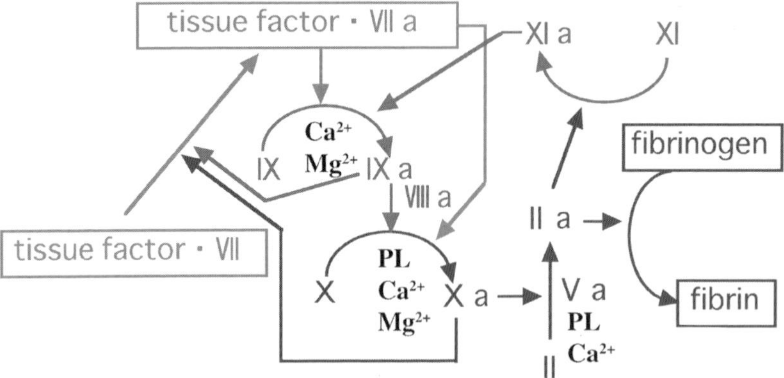

Fig. 1. Blood coagulation cascade.

The hepatic sinusoid is a unique microcirculation system in blood coagulation as well as in structure. In the hepatic sinusoids, Kupffer cells exist as resident macrophages and endothelial cells show no expression of TFPI [4] and minimal expression of thrombomodulin [5,6]. This may imply that microcirculatory disturbance due to sinusoidal fibrin deposition can develop easily when tissue factor activity is increased on Kupffer cells after activation. According to our observations, such a disturbance can cause massive liver necrosis in rats which are given endotoxin following heat-killed *Propionibacterium acnes* pretreatment or 70% partial hepatectomy [5,7—11] and undergo orthotopic liver transplantation

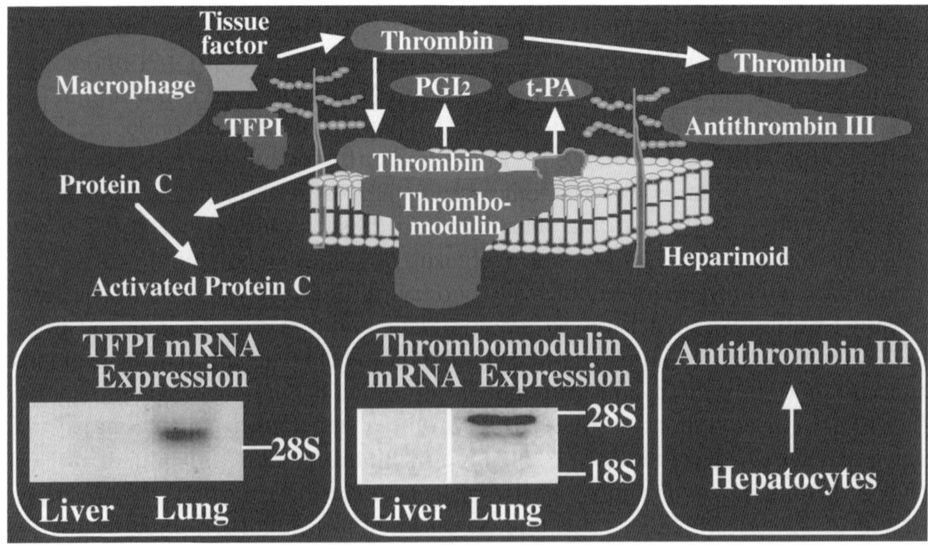

Fig. 2. Anticoagulant factors on vascular endothelial cells.

[6,12−15]. Similar mechanisms seem to contribute to the development of fulminant viral hepatitis and liver injury after cadaveric liver transplantation in humans [12,16,17]. Thus, blood coagulation disorder is an important contributing factor to acute liver failure in liver diseases.

DIC (disseminated intravascular coagulation) in liver cirrhosis

In cirrhotic liver, capillarization of the hepatic sinusoids occurs in association with extracellular matrix deposition produced by activated stellate cells in the space of Disse [18]. Capillarized endothelial cells in rats with liver cirrhosis show increased thrombomodulin expression compared to sinusoidal endothelial cells in normal rats [5], suggesting that antithrombogenic function may be more active in cirrhotic liver than in normal liver. However, thrombomodulin mRNA expression examined by Northern blot analysis is much smaller even in cirrhotic liver than in other organs such as the lung. Moreover, hepatic macrophages isolated from cirrhotic liver show higher tissue factor activity compared to Kupffer cells from normal liver [5]. Thus, blood coagulopathy can develop easily in cirrhotic liver, when Kupffer cells and hepatic macrophages become activated to express tissue factor abundantly (Fig. 3).

Blood coagulation factors except for tissue factor and factor VIII are produced exclusively by hepatocytes. Hepatocytes produce anticoagulant factors such as antithrombin (AT) III, a serine protease inhibitor which can induce irreversible inactivation of thrombin by forming thrombin-AT III complex (TAT) [19]. Thus, the amounts of both thrombogenic and antithrombogenic factors are small in the plasma of advanced liver cirrhosis patients, suggesting that blood coagulation imbalance can easily occur in response to increased tissue factor activity (Fig. 4). In these patients, chronic compensated DIC state is suggested to exist universally [20], since the clearance rate of tissue factor and activated coagulation fac-

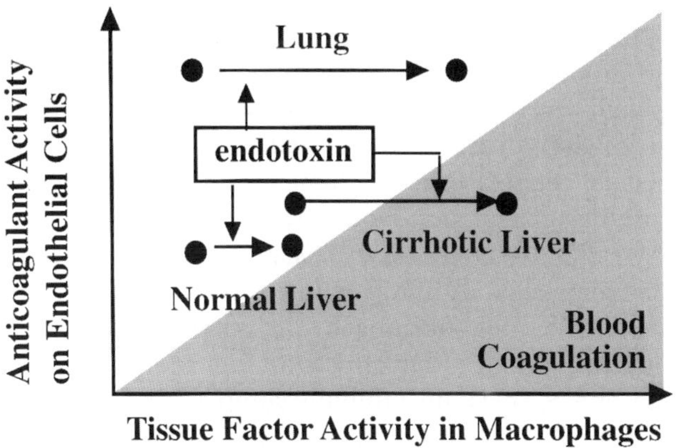

Fig. 3. Blood coagulation equilibrium in the peripheral vessels.

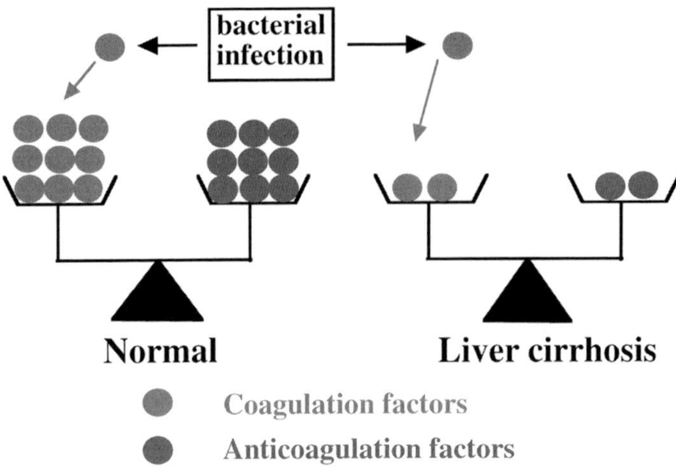

Fig. 4. Blood coagulation equilibrium in the plasma.

tors from the circulation is reduced as a result of impaired phagocytotic function of Kupffer cells [21]. Furthermore, acute fulminant DIC is shown to develop frequently in these patients after bacterial infection or treatment with peritoneal venous (LeVeen) shunts [22]. Thus, DIC is a commonly observed complication which may affect the prognosis of liver cirrhosis patients through provocation of general bleeding tendency.

Diagnosis of DIC in liver cirrhosis

In Japan, DIC is generally diagnosed according to the criteria proposed by the Blood Coagulation Disorders Study Group, Ministry of Health and Welfare in 1988. According to these criteria, the diagnosis is made based on peripheral platelet count, prothrombin time and plasma concentrations of fibrinogen and fibrin/fibrinogen degradation products (FDP). These criteria are useful for the diagnosis of DIC in patients with sepsis and malignant diseases. However, their utility is limited in the case of liver diseases. Liver cirrhosis patients usually show decreased peripheral platelet counts due to hypersplenism caused by portal hypertension. Fibrinogen as well as coagulation factors II, V, VII and X are produced exclusively by hepatocytes, and thereby their plasma concentrations and prothrombin time are deranged in patients with liver failure without complication of DIC. In cirrhotic patients with ascites, fibrinogen in peritoneal effusion is degraded to form FDP and increase plasma FDP concentration. Molecular markers such as TAT and plasmin and α2 plasmin inhibitor complex (PIC) are not useful; the increase of both complex concentrations in the plasma is minimal even when DIC develops [17], because AT III and α2 plasmin inhibitor are less produced by hepatocytes.

In this situation, serial measurements of peripheral platelet count are the most useful for early diagnosis of DIC. When peripheral platelet count is progressively decreased, attention should be paid to the development of DIC. The presence of DIC is also possible when the derangements of prothrombin time and plasma fibrinogen concentration are exacerbated with no changes in serum concentrations of cholinesterase and bilirubin. In such cases, the diagnosis of DIC can be made if plasma TAT concentration is markedly increased after intravenous infusion of AT III concentrate, since this increase reflects excessive thrombin present in the plasma [17]. It is reported that plasma concentration of prothrombin fragment 1+2 is a marker more sensitive than plasma TAT concentration for detecting hypercoagulopathy [23]. Plasma concentration of factors VIII:C and VIII:R is produced by endothelial cells, but not by hepatocytes [24]. The usefulness of these markers is to be elucidated.

Treatment of DIC in liver cirrhosis

When DIC is suspected by a gradual decrease of peripheral platelet count in patients with liver cirrhosis, continuous infusion of synthetic protease inhibitors should be started. For this purpose, gabexate mesilate and nafamostat mesilate are available in Japan. Both agents inhibit the actions of activated coagulation factors independently of AT III [25]. In addition, gabexate mesilate can attenuate fibrinolysis [26], and nafamostat mesilate can suppress cytokine and superoxide release from monocytes and neutrophils [27]. Thus, these inhibitors are preferable in the treatment of DIC especially initiated by bacterial infection in cirrhotic patients. Antibiotic therapy can also attenuate such DIC.

AT III concentrate is intravenously injected when the efficacy of synthetic protease inhibitors is minimal or the progression of DIC is rash in cirrhotic patients. Use of heparin and low-molecular-weight heparin, cofactors of AT III [28], should be avoided unless plasma AT III concentration is maintained higher than 80% of normal levels after administration of AT III concentrate and synthetic protease inhibitors, because plasma AT III concentration is markedly consumed, and such consumption of AT III can exacerbate DIC in rat models of liver failure [7].

For the treatment of fibrin deposition in the hepatic sinusoids, supplementation of TFPI and thrombomodulin, targeting the sinusoidal walls, would be a promising strategy. When rh-TFPI is intravenously injected in rats, it disappears rapidly from the circulation, but is detected by electron microscopy on the surface of sinusoidal endothelial cells and microvilli of hepatocytes in the space of Disse [4]. This TFPI reappears in the circulation after an intravenous injection of heparin, showing its reduced immunohistochemical stains on the hepatic sinusoidal walls (Fig. 5) [4], suggesting that exogenous TFPI can increase anticoagulant activity exclusively on the hepatic sinusoidal walls by binding to heparinoids on the cell surface. Moreover, it is noteworthy that this treatment can increase anticoagulant activity on the hepatic sinusoids even when endothelial cells are lost [29].

82

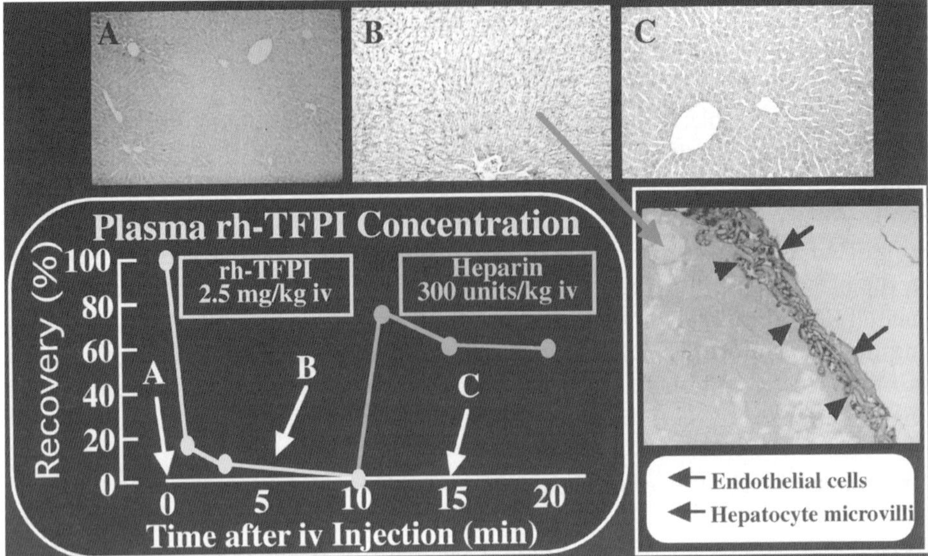

Fig. 5. Immunohistochemical staining of TFPI in rat liver.

Attenuation of activation of Kupffer cells and hepatic macrophages may be effective for the prevention of DIC in liver cirrhosis patients. For patients with liver cirrhosis, intestinal wall congestion caused by portal hypertension may increase bacterial translocation from the gut to the portal blood. According to our observation, the overloading of gut-derived substances can increase tissue factor activity in Kupffer cells in rats [6]. When rats receive oral administration of polymyxin B sulfate for 7 days, bacterial flora are significantly altered in the gut; *Enterobacteriaceae* diminish and anaerobes such as *Bifidobacterium* and *Lactobacillus* increase in number [15]. This treatment can also reduce endotoxin concentration in the portal blood 30 mins following blood reflow after portal vein occlusion [15]. In orthotopic liver transplantation, the increase of tissue factor activity in Kupffer cells in recipient rats is markedly reduced by pretreatment with polymyxin B sulfate with attenuation of liver necrosis at 24 h after the operation [15]. Polymyxin B sulfate would be also effective for prevention against DIC in liver cirrhosis patients.

References

1. Nemerson Y. Tissue factor and hemostasis. Blood 1988;71:1—8.
2. Esmon CT. The role of protein C and thrombomodulin in the regulation of blood coagulation. J Biol Chem 1989;17:4743—4746.
3. Broze GJ Jr. Tissue factor pathway inhibitor and the current concept of blood coagulation. Blood Coag Fibrinol 1995;6:S7—S13.
4. Yamanobe F, Mochida S, Ohno A, Ishikawa K, Fujiwara K. Recombinant human tissue factor pathway inhibitor as a possible anticoagulant targeting hepatic sinusoidal walls. Thromb Res

1997;85:493—501.

5. Arai M, Mochida S, Ohno A, Ogata I, Obama H, Maruyama I, Fujiwara K. Blood coagulation equilibrium in rat liver microcirculation as evaluated by endothelial cell thrombomodulin and macrophage tissue factor. Thromb Res 1995;80:113—123.

6. Arai M, Mochida S, Ohno A, Kurokawa K, Fujiwara K. Coagulability in the sinusoids of orthotopically transplanted livers in rats. Transpl Proc 1994;26:913—915.

7. Yamada S, Ogata I, Hirata K, Mochida S, Tomiya T, Fujiwara K. Intravascular coagulation in the development of massive hepatic necrosis induced by Corynebacterium parvum and endotoxin in rats. Scand J Gastroenterol 1989;24:293—298.

8. Mochida S, Ogata I, Hirata K, Ohta Y, Yamada S, Fujiwara K. Provocation of massive hepatic necrosis by endotoxin after partial hepatectomy in rats. Gastroenterology 1990;99:771—777.

9. Arai M, Mochida S, Ohno A, Ogata I, Fujiwara K. Sinusoidal endothelial cell damage by activated macrophages in rat liver necrosis. Gastroenterology 1993;104:1466—1471.

10. Mochida S, Ohno A, Arai M, Fujiwara K. The role of adhesion between activated macrophages and endothelial cells in the development of two types of massive hepatic necrosis in rats. J Gastroenterol Hepatol 1995;10:S38—S42.

11. Mochida S, Ohno A, Arai M, Tamatani T, Miyasaka M, Fujiwara K. Role of adhesion molecules in the development of massive hepatic necrosis in rats. Hepatology 1996;23:320—328.

12. Fujiwara K, Mochida S, Arai M, Ohno A. Possible causes of primary graft nonfunction after orthotopic liver transplantation: a hypothesis with rat models. J Gastroenterol Hepatol 1995; 10:S88—S91.

13. Arai M, Mochida S, Ohno A, Fujiwara K. Blood coagulation in the hepatic sinusoids as a contributing factor of liver injury following orthotopic liver transplantation in rats. Transplantation 1996;62:1398—1401.

14. Mochida S, Arai M, Ohno A, Fujiwara K. Bacterial translocation from gut to portal blood as a factor of hypercoagulopathy in the hepatic sinusoids after orthotopic liver transplantation in rats. Transpl Proc 1997;29:874—875.

15. Arai M, Nochida S, Ohno A, Arai S, Fujiwara K. Selective bowel decontamination of recipients for prevention against liver injury following orthotopic liver transplantation: evaluation with rat models. Hepatology 1998;27:123—127.

16. Fujiwara K, Okita K, Akamatsu K, Abe H, Tameda Y, Sakai T, Inoue N, Kanai K, Aoki N, Oka H. Antithrombin III concentrate in the treatment of fulminant hepatic failure. Gastroenterol Jpn 1988;23:423—427.

17. Tomiya T, Ogata I, Fujiwara K. Inhibition of thrombin generation in fulminanthepatic failure by treatment with antithrombin III. Biomed Prog 1989;3:39—40.

18. Shaffner F, Popper H. Capillarization of hepatic sinusoids in man. Gastroenterology 1963;44: 239—242.

19. Downing MR, Bloom JW, Mann KG. Comparison of the inhibition of thrombin by three plasma protease inhibitors. Biochemistry 1978;17:2649—2653.

20. Schipper HG, TenCate JW. Antithrombin III transfusion in patients with hepatic cirrhosis. Br J Haematol 1982;52:25—33.

21. Verstraete M, Vermylen J, Collen D. Intravascular coagulation in liver disease. Ann Rev Med 1974;25:447—452.

22. Salem HH, Dudley FJ, Merrett A, Perkin J, Firkin BG. Coagulopathy of peritonealveous shunts: studies on pathologic role of ascitic fluid collagen and value of antiplatelet therapy. Gut 1983; 24:412—417.

23. Takahashi H, Wada K, Niwano H, Shibata A. Comparison of prothrombin fragment 1+2 with thrombin-antithrombin III complex in plasma of patients with disseminated intravascular coagulation. Blood Coag Fibrinol 1992;3:813—818.

24. Hirata K, Ogata I, Ohta Y, Fujiwara K. Hepatic sinusoidal destruction in the development of intravascular coagulation in acute liver failure of rats. J Pathol 1989;158:157—165.

25. Ohno H, Kambayashi J, Chang SW, Kosaki G. FOY: (Ethyl p-{6-uanidinohexanoyloxy}benzo-

ate) methanesulfonate as a serine protease inhibitor. I. Inhibition of thrombin and factor Xa in vitro. Thromb Res 1980;19:579—588.

26. Tamura Y, Hirano M, Okamura K, Minato Y, Fujii S. Synthetic inhibitors of trypsin, plasmin, kakkikrein, thrombin, C1r- and C1 esterase. Biochem Biophys Acta 1977;484:417—422.

27. Suzuki M, Suematsu M, Miura S, Oshio C, Oda M, Tsuchiya M. Microcirculatory disturbances in endotoxin-induced disseminated intravascular coagulation. The effects of heparin and gabexate mesilate on locomotive and metabolic changes of neutrophils. Adv Exp Med Biol 1988;242: 135—141.

28. Rosenberg RD, Damus PS. The purification and mechanisms of action of human antithrombin-heparin cofactor. J Biol Chem 1973;248:6490—6505.

29. Mochida S, Arai S, Yamanobe F, Ohno A, Kato H, Fujiwara K. Anticoagulant targeting for hepatic sinusoidal walls in prevention of hypercoagulopathy in cold preserved rat livers. Transpl Proc 1998;30:45—48.

Progress in Hepatology, Volume 4.
Liver Cirrhosis Update.
M. Yamanaka et al., editors.

85

Impaired glucose tolerance in liver cirrhosis

Teruji Tanaka

Department of Internal Medicine (I), Daisan Hospital, Jikei University School of Medicine, Tokyo

Abstract. Liver dysfunction, especially liver cirrhosis, is often associated with glucose intolerance and the pathogenesis of this metabolic disorder has been investigated extensively. There is still no consensus regarding its mechanism. In clinical settings we often encounter diabetic conditions in patients with liver cirrhosis, so-called hepatogenic diabetes. Such diabetes should be differentiated from primary diabetes. Our studies, described here, show several distinctive differences between the diabetic states, including the effect on arteriosclerosis, galactose metabolism and prognosis. Further, since glucose intolerance in cirrhosis is currently thought to be associated with insulin resistance which is probably associated with a combination of insulin receptor binding and postbinding defects, our group have recently focused on investigating insulin receptor substrate-1, being one of the possible candidate proteins associated with insulin resistance in liver cirrhosis. It is important to figure out, in clinical settings, whether the diabetic condition in cirrhosis could be treated as general diabetes with significant hyperglycemia and several complications.

Keywords: arteriosclerosis, diabetes mellitus, galactose, glucose intolerance, insulin receptor substrate-1, liver cirrhosis.

Introduction

It is widely known that the liver plays an important role in carbohydrate homeostasis, and an enormous number of investigations have demonstrated a high frequency of abnormal carbohydrate tolerance, along with a state of insulin resistance, in patients with impaired liver function. Furthermore, liver disease-associated diabetes mellitus has been discussed by many investigators, since diabetes mellitus is known to be a common complication of chronic liver damage. Therefore, the association between the two clinical conditions, liver disease and diabetes, is very complex and problematic. The association in terms of first cause and biochemical and physiological nature still remains obscure.

Diabetes as a consequence of liver disease, the so-called hepatogenic diabetes, was first recognized early in the 20th century. In 1906, Naunyn pointed out that liver cirrhosis is often associated with glucose intolerance [1]. Taub et al. [2] classified hyperglycemic patients into the following three groups: 1) actual insulin deficiency is due to malfunction of the islets of Langerhans in the pancreas, 2) relative insulin deficiency is due primarily to an excessive production of the pituitary and adrenal gland hormones which regulate carbohydrate metabolism, 3) one of the most frequent manifestations of hepatic insufficiency is the inability

Address for correspondence: Prof Teruji Tanaka MD, Department of Internal Medicine (I), Daisan Hospital, Jikei University School of Medicine, 4-11-1 Izumihonchyo, Komae City, Tokyo 201, Japan.

to regulate the blood glucose properly. They then suggested that the dysfunction in the majority of adult-onset primary diabetes mellitus was hepatic rather than pancreatic in origin. Indeed, therapy directed toward the liver has been shown to achieve far greater success in the management of the hepatogenic diabetic patients compared to insulin administration and a diabetic regimen. Leevy et al. [3] suggested that liver abnormalities frequently cause hyperglycemia and glucosuria and stressed the importance of early recognition and proper treatment of hepatogenic diabetes. Their view is supported by the observation of transient hyperglycemia in patients with fatty liver, hepatitis, and biliary infection. In Japan, Takahashi et al. [4] argued against the concept of the so-called hepatogenic diabetes and stated their understanding that hepatogenic diabetes is one of the metabolic patterns manifested as a consequence of liver dysfunction. In 1969, Conn et al. [5] studied the frequency of diabetes, defined as persistent fasting hyperglycemia, in a group of 240 consecutive cirrhotic patients and a control group of 411 randomly selected, age-matched noncirrhotic patients, and showed that a diabetic state was significantly more common in the cirrhotic group (16.7%) than in the noncirrhotic group (7.1%), and that cirrhosis was apparent before diabetes was detected in most of the subjects (diabetes was diagnosed first in 18%). After more than two decades, there is still no consensus on the mechanisms of derangement of glucose metabolism in patients with cirrhosis, although many studies have been published from the viewpoints of insulin action, insulin receptor and insulin resistance [6–8].

In this paper, derangement of glucose metabolism in the patients with chronic liver diseases, especially cirrhosis, is discussed, based on the condensed data from our department.

Glucose intolerance and insulin response to a glucose load in cirrhotic patients

The pathogenesis of glucose intolerance accompanying cirrhosis is intriguing. Cirrhotic patients in general show hyperinsulinemia and exaggerated insulin release in response to a glucose load [6–9]. In a previous study conducted in our department [10], 210 patients with chronic liver diseases were divided into three groups based on OGTT results according to the guidelines of the Japanese Association of Diabetes Mellitus [11]; diabetic response group (n = 71), borderline response group (n = 105) and normal response group (n = 34). As shown in Table 1, the majority of the patients with liver damage demonstrated a diabetic pattern in OGTT. The proportions of the diabetic response group plus the borderline response group were 75.8% in acute hepatitis, 80.8% in chronic hepatitis, 81.7% in precirrhosis and 94.7% in cirrhosis. Furthermore, 56.1% of cirrhotic patients with low values of indocyanine green test (K < 0.100) showed a diabetic response in OGTT. Among the cirrhotic patients, 50.6% demonstrated a diabetic response in OGTT, which was a significantly higher (p < 0.01) incidence than those with other patterns of response (36.1% for borderline and 13.3% for normal response). Such cirrhotic patients showed hypersecretion of insulin as well

Table 1. Patterns of glucose tolerance test results and characteristics of liver disease.

Types of disease	No. of patients	Glucose tolerance test (% in parentheses)		
		Normal	Borderline	Diabetic
Fatty liver	40	5 (12.5)	22 (55)	13 (32.5)
Acute hepatitis	29	7 (24.5)	20 (68.9)	2 (6.9)
Chronic hepatitis	47	9 (19.2)	26 (55.3)	12 (25.5)
Pre-Cirrhosis	11	2 (18.2)	7 (63.6)	2 (18.2)
Cirrhosis	83	11 (13.3)	30 (36.1)	42 (50.6)
$ICG_K > 0.101$	42	5 (11.9)	18 (42.8)	19 (45.2)
$ICG_K \leqslant 0.100$	41	6 (14.6)	12 (29.3)	29 (56.1)

Total 210 cases; ICG_K = indocyanine green test.

as a diabetic profile of blood glucose in OGTT as shown in Fig. 1.

In our other study [11] examining the insulinogenic index (calculated by change in immunoreactive insulin/change in blood glucose (IRI/BS) at 30 min postload of glucose), which is a reliable marker of insulin secretion [12], the mean value of the index was higher in patients with chronic hepatitis (0.88) and cirrhosis (1.75) than in those with primary diabetes mellitus (0.21) (Fig. 2A). It is noteworthy that there were some cases of cirrhosis with indices similar to primary diabetic cases. Such patients may have an impairment of pancreatic endogenous hormonal function. Next, we investigated the hypersecreting state of insulin during glucose load in patients with hepatogenic diabetes. The summation of blood glucose level (BS) $\Sigma BS^{180'}$ and that of immunoreactive insulin (IRI) $\Sigma IRI^{180'}$ were calculated by totalling the levels from predose to 180 min postdose. From the relationship between $\Sigma BS^{180'}$ and $\Sigma IRI^{180'}$ shown in Fig. 3, $\Sigma BS^{180'}$ increases with the elevation of $\Sigma IRI^{180'}$ in most cirrhotic patients, while $\Sigma BS^{180'}$ increase is not accompanied by $\Sigma IRI^{180'}$ increase in patients with diabetes mellitus. The $\Sigma IRI^{180'}/\Sigma BS^{180'}$ ratio differentiates clearly between hepatogenic diabetes and primary diabetes mellitus (Fig. 2B); the mean ratios were 0.054 in cirrhotic patients and 0.047 in controls, which were significantly higher than that in patients with primary diabetes mellitus (0.016). The cirrhotic patients exhibited a wide range of $\Sigma IRI^{180'}/\Sigma BS^{180'}$ ratio; some cases had high ratios above 0.075 which demonstrated insulin hypersecretion, whilst others had low values below 0.002 as observed in primary diabetes mellitus.

Alcohol intake and glucose intolerance

Chronic consumption of ethanol is known to be associated with pancreatic injury as well as hepatic damage [3,13]. It is obscure how chronic consumption of

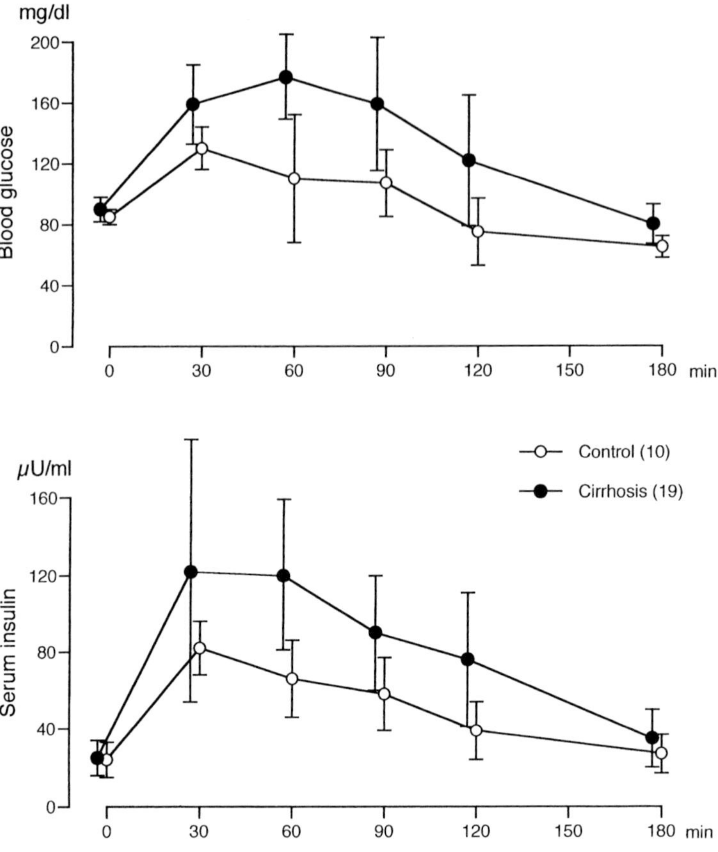

Fig. 1. Blood glucose and serum insulin levels in oral glucose tolerance test in patients with cirrhosis and controls. Open circles indicate the values of controls; closed circles indicate values of cirrhotic subjects.

ethanol modifies insulin secretion in patients with chronic liver diseases. Our group investigated the average daily alcohol intake/total alcohol intake in 47 patients with chronic hepatitis and 97 patients with cirrhosis. Figure 4A shows that the mean daily alcohol intake was 74.1 g in chronic hepatitis patients and 101.6 g in cirrhotic patients. The average daily alcohol intake was greater in the diabetic response group than in the other groups (borderline response and normal response groups) for both cirrhotic and chronic hepatitis patients. Furthermore, the total alcohol intake was greater (around 550 kg) in the diabetic response group in chronic hepatitis patients and in the borderline response and diabetic response groups in cirrhotic patients compared to the other groups (Fig. 4B). However, since the cirrhotic patients with high alcohol intake showed hypersecretion of insulin in OGTT and high value of insulinogenic index in this investigation, alcohol-related hepatic injury does not appear to be related to the impairment of insulin secretion from the pancreas.

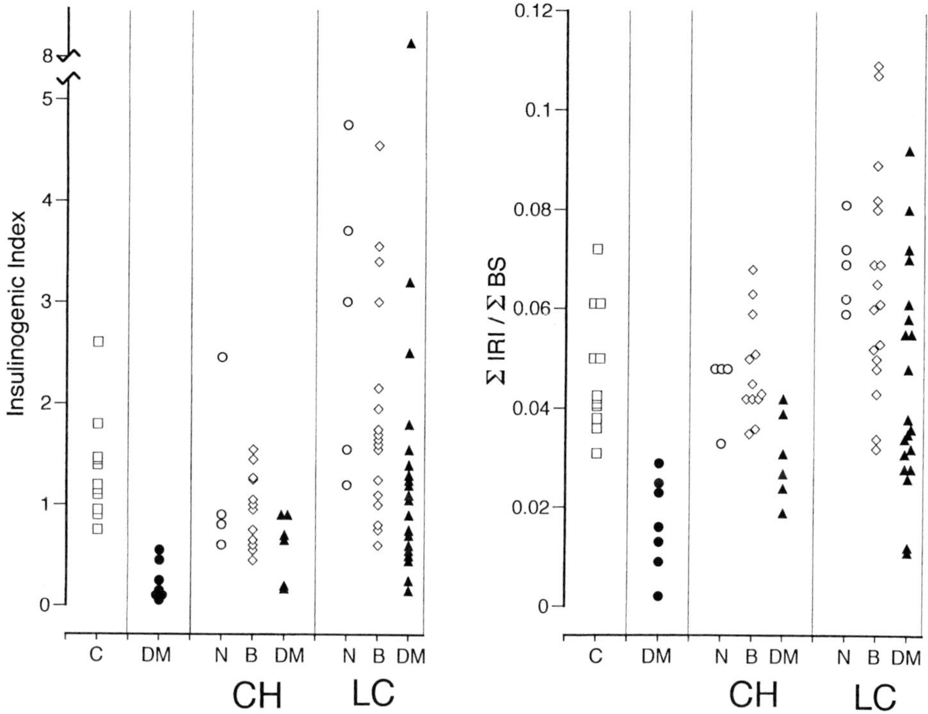

Fig. 2. Left panel (A): insulinogenic index (IRI/BS 30′) after oral glucose load in patients with chronic liver diseases. Right panel (B): ΣIRI/ΣBS after oral glucose load in patients with chronic liver diseases. IRI = immunoreactive insulin (μu/ml), BS = blood glucose (mg/dl), CH = chronic hepatitis, LC = liver cirrhosis, DM = diabetes mellitus, □: normal control (C), ●: primary diabetes (DM), ○: normal response (N), ◇: borderline response (B), ▲: diabetic response (DM).

Hepatogenic diabetes and arteriosclerosis

Empirical clinical experience and several clinical investigations have shown that cirrhotic condition in the liver ameliorates systemic arteriosclerosis, and such patients have been reported to be less complicated with systemic hypertension [14–17]. On the other hand, sclerotic changes in arterioles is known to be accelerated in patients with diabetes mellitus. Most of the advance cirrhotic patients have poor glucose tolerance and unstable blood glucose levels clinically. To investigate amelioration or acceleration of arteriosclerosis, our group conducted microscopic examinations of coronary and renal arterioles in 39 autopsy cases with only liver cirrhosis, 22 cases with cirrhosis and a diabetes state and 54 age-matched control patients [17]. The ratio of the arteriole lumen (S) to total arteriole area (L) was used as an index for arteriosclerotic change. As shown in Fig. 5, the presence of a cirrhotic condition (LC), even combined with a diabetes state (LC+DM), ameliorated the coronary arteriosclerotic change in both the older

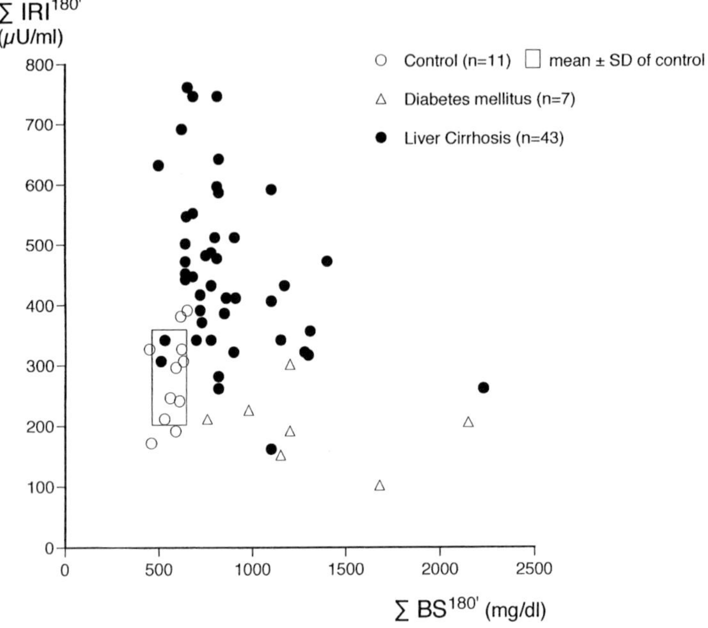

Fig. 3. The relationship between $\Sigma BS^{180'}$ and $\Sigma IRI^{180'}$ in an oral glucose tolerance test over 180 min. Rectangle indicates Mean ± SD value of the control. IRI = immunoreactive insulin (µu/ml), BS = blood glucose (mg/dl), $\Sigma X^{180'}$ = summation of all values from predose to 180 min postdose.

group (≥ 60 years) and the younger group (≤ 60 years) (p < 005), and an amelioration of arteriosclerotic change was also observed in the renal arterioles in cirrhotic patients in both age groups.

Hepatogenic diabetes and diabetic retinopathy

Vascular retinopathy is a frequent complication of diabetes mellitus and the progress has recently been reported to be associated with a long diabetic duration and high blood glucose level [18—20]. Recently our group analyzed the grade of diabetic retinopathy (Fukuda classification: A_0, A_{1-2}; nonproliferative, and B_1; proliferative retinopathy) in 53 cases with cirrhosis and a diabetic state, and compared them with 230 control cases with only diabetes mellitus. We also investigated plasma glycosylated hemoglobin level (HbA1c) in both groups. As shown in Table 2, the duration of disease and HbA1c level were similar in both groups. The frequency of development of each stage of retinopathy was also similar in both groups. These findings suggest that a diabetic condition manifested as high blood glucose level is an important deleterious factor in the development of diabetic retinopathy. These findings are in agreement with the recent concept that diabetic retinopathy appears to be caused only by a high blood glucose condition and not by other diabetic metabolic characteristics [21,22].

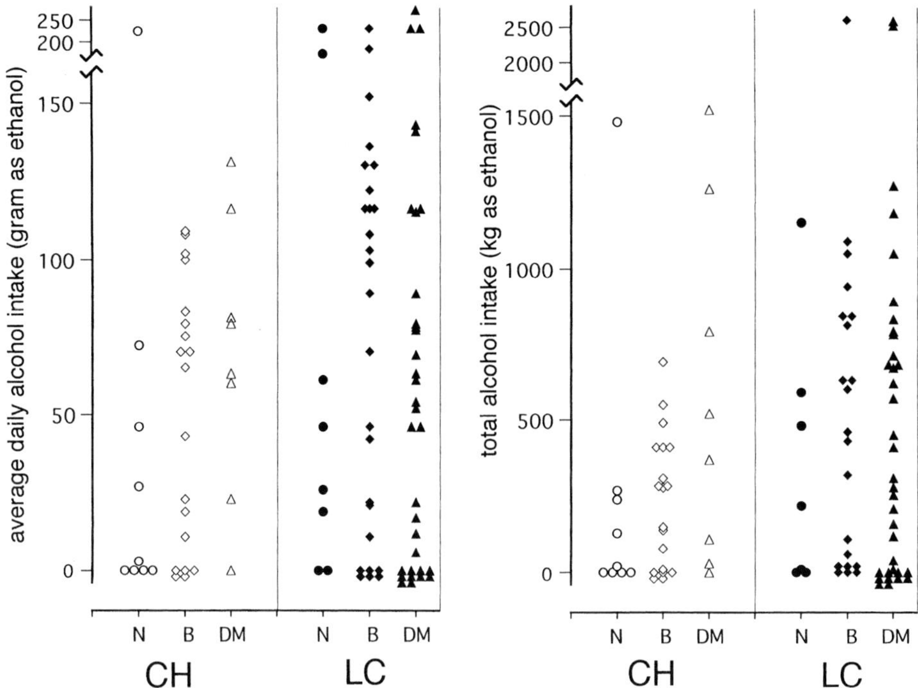

Fig. 4. Relationship between average (left panel — A) and total (right panel — B) alcohol intake and patterns of glucose tolerance test in patients with chronic hepatitis and cirrhosis. CH = chronic hepatitis, LC = liver cirrhosis, $\bigcirc$, $\bullet$: normal response (N), $\diamond$, $\blacklozenge$: borderline response (B), $\triangle$, $\blacktriangle$: diabetic response (DM).

Galactose challenge test in chronic liver diseases

Galactose is utilized mainly in the liver for the biosynthesis of glucose, and is converted into glucose and metabolized through the glycolysis pathway. Galactose tolerance test (GaTT) has been used as a hepatic function test to evaluate the galactose metabolic ability [23,24]. When insulin secretion is not impaired,

Table 2. Grade of diabetic retinopathy and clinical characteristics in patients with cirrhosis and diabetes or primary diabetes mellitus.

Fukuda's grade	Cirrhosis with diabetes			Diabetes mellitus		
	A_0	A_{1-2}	B_1	A_0	A_{1-2}	B_1
Disease year	5.4 ± 1.2	6.4 ± 1.2	16^a	5.5 ± 0.6	8.1 ± 0.7	9.7 ± 0.8
Frequency	60	38	2	64	21	7
HbA_{1c}	9.1 ± 0.5	8.9 ± 0.7	13.8^a	9.6 ± 0.1	10.2 ± 0.2	9.2 ± 0.3

Fukuda classification: A_0, A_{1-2}; nonproliferative, and B_1; proliferative retinopathy. [a]Data from one patient.

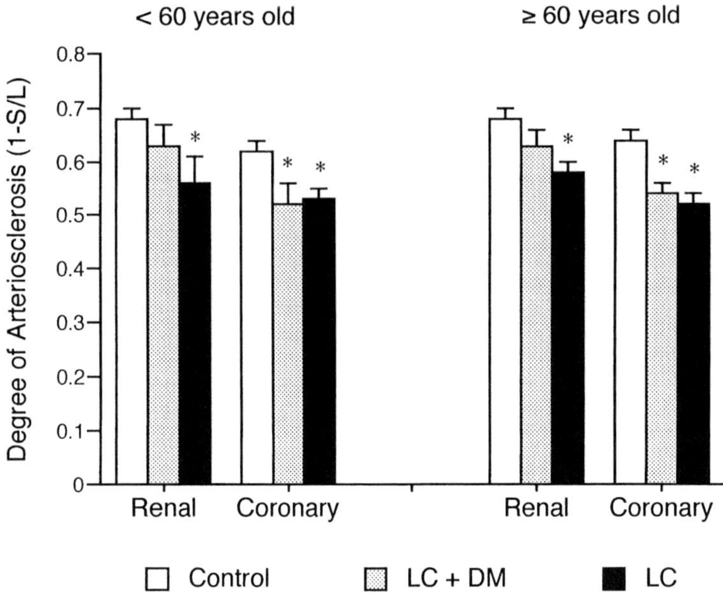

Fig. 5. The age-related degree of arteriosclerosis $(1-S/L)$ in renal and coronary arteriole in patients with cirrhosis (LC) with or without diabetes (DM) and in controls. Where S is arteriole lumen and L is total arteriole area. Open bar indicates the mean value of controls, hatched bar indicates the mean value of cirrhosis complicated with diabetes and closed bar indicates the mean value of cirrhosis. $*p < 0.05$ compared with the control.

the plasma glucose response with time, following a galactose load, is known to be flat. This contrast with cases when insulin secretion is impaired, since the production of glucose from galactose is accelerated by enhanced glycogenesis and glycogen degradation, and suppressed glycolysis and glycogen biosynthesis. In this case, the plasma glucose response with time, following a galactose load, is a curve which is variably dependent on liver function. Our group investigated the glucose response following a 40 g oral galactose load in patients with chronic liver diseases (n = 72) (cirrhosis and chronic hepatitis) and patients with diabetes mellitus and no liver damage (n = 19) [25]. Patients with chronic liver diseases were further divided in two groups by the value of $\Delta IRI/\Delta BS$ (index of insulin secretion; cut off point 0.4) [12]. A value below 0.4 is known to indicate poor insulin secretion. Table 3 demonstrates that the plasma glucose increase after a galactose load was small in the group with indices over 0.4, while the increase in the group with indices below 0.4 was more than twofold that of the former group. As shown in Table 3, blood glucose increase at 30 min after a galactose load is a reasonable marker to use to differentiate between the groups with (11.6 $\pm$ 6.4) and without chronic liver diseases (25.4 $\pm$ 8.5) for patients with indices below 0.4. We also investigated the relationship between the plasma glucose and galactose levels following a 40 g oral galactose load in patients with chronic liver

Table 3. Comparison of change in blood glucose level after 40 g oral galactose load in patients with various conditions of liver diseases.

$\Delta IRI/\Delta BS_{30\,min}$ in 50 g OGTT	Subjects	No. of patients	Δglucose in GaTT (mg/dl)	
			30 min	120 min
Below 0.4	Diabetes without liver diseases	19	25.4 ± 8.5	20.3 ± 14.3 20.4 ± 14.3^a
	Chronic liver disease	20	11.6 ± 6.4	20.6 ± 16.4
Above 0.4	Chronic liver diseases	52	4.3 ± 4.7	2.6 ± 5.3

Data are presented as mean $\pm$ SD. [a]Mean $\pm$ SD of Glucose in all subjects with $IRI/BS_{30\,min}$ below 0.4.

diseases who had $\Delta IRI/\Delta BS$ indices below 0.4 (Fig. 6). The patients were made up of 15 with liver cirrhosis, 4 with chronic hepatitis, and 19 with primary dia-

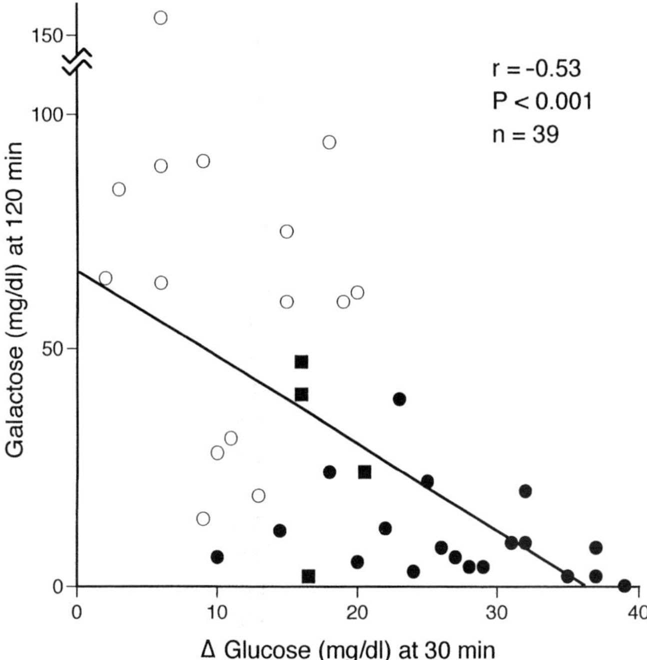

Fig. 6. The relationship between galactose level at 120 min postload and change of glucose level at 30 min postload after a 40 g oral galactose load in patients with chronic liver diseases who had $\Delta IRI/\Delta BS$ indices below 0.4. A significant inverse correlation (r $= -0.53$, p < 0.001) was observed. ●: primary diabetes, ■: chronic hepatitis, ○: cirrhosis.

betes mellitus. The value of Δglucose at 30 min following a galactose load correlates inversely with the galactose value at 120 min and this correlation is statistically significant ($p < 0.001$). The diabetic and cirrhotic subjects occupy the lower right part and the upper left part of the graph, respectively. This relationship suggests that the value of Δglucose at 30 min following a galactose load reflects the liver function as galactose metabolic ability well, and that a galactose load test can be a useful method for assessing patients with various liver diseases — one aspect of the liver metabolic functions.

Insulin secretion and prognosis in cirrhotic patients

Fasting hyperinsulinemia has been described in patients with various degrees of cirrhosis. In patients with liver disease, decreased degradation of insulin by the liver has been suggested to be the principal cause of hyperinsulinemia. However, various issues remain unsolved, such as how impaired liver function influences the degree of insulin secretion and degradation as well as fasting insulin/glucose level in blood, and whether insulin response in OGTT predicts the degree of liver function impairment and ultimately the prognosis of cirrhotic patients [26–28]. Against this background, our group investigated the relationship between fasting plasma glucose level and insulin secreting ability in OGTT [29]. We also examined the incidence of hepatic encephalopathy and the prognosis in cirrhotic patients (n = 145) [29]. As shown in Table 4, the group of diabetic patients with high fasting plasma glucose levels (FPG) (> 140 mg/dl) secreted insulin poorly, while diabetic patients with low-FPG (< 140 mg/dl) and nondiabetic cirrhotic patients secreted insulin normally. However, diabetic patients, both with high- and low-FPG, had a significantly higher incidence of encephalopathy and mortality than the nondiabetic group. Diabetic patients with low-FPG group and a greater than 2.5-fold increase of FPG at 2-h OGTT had severe liver damage and poor prognosis ($p < 0.0.1$, Table 4). These results suggest that in cirrhotic patients with severe damage, a markedly decreased glycogen store and impaired glyconeogenesis in liver may induce relative hypoglycemia, and impaired glycolysis and glycogen biosynthesis may trigger hyperglycemia after a glucose load.

Table 4. Insulin secretion and prognosis in patients with cirrhosis.

75 g OGTT pattern	No. of patients	Insulin secretion impairment (%)	Hepatic encephalopathy (%)	Mortality (%)
Nondiabetic	(66)	5	3	0
Diabetic				
FPG ⩽ 140 mg/dl	(29)	88	18	7
FPG > 140 mg/dl				
group 1	(25)	16	18	0
group 2	(25)	16	86	48

FPG = fasting plasma glucose. Group 1: 2 h value/FPG < 2.5, group 2: 2 h value/FPG $\geqslant 2.5$.

Cirrhosis and sensitivity of insulin receptor

Insulin binding to a specific receptor regulates cellular growth and metabolism through activation of the tyrosine kinase in the receptor. Insulin-stimulated receptor autophosphorylation activates the tyrosine kinase domain in the cytosol, leading to tyrosine phosphorylation of the endogenous substrates that are thought to play important roles in signal transmission as second messenger molecules. Insulin receptor substrate-1 (IRS-1), which was first reported by White et al. [30] as a pp185 protein is the major cellular substrate for insulin receptor b-subunit tyrosine kinase. Nishiyama et al. [31] isolated IRS-1 genomic DNA from a human placental genomic library. The structure of IRS-1 shows it is a unique molecule containing multiple phosphorylation sites including nine potential tyrosine phosphorylation motifs YMXM and YXXM (where Y and M refer to tyrosine and methionine, respectively) which are excellent substrates for tyrosine kinase of the insulin receptor b-subunit as well as insulin-like growth factor I (IGF-1). Following tyrosine phosphorylation, these motifs bind to molecules containing the Src-homology domains 2 and 3, such as phosphatidyl inositol-3 kinase, SHPTP-2, and growth factor receptor bound-2 [32]. Recent study [33] revealed that IRS-1 is one of the intracellular substrates for interleukin-4 (IL-4) and participates in the IL-4 signaling pathways.

We isolated the human IRS-1 genomic DNA as well as identifying the chromosomal localization of the human IRS-1 gene, and developed a fluorescence in situ hybridization technique using a genomic DNA clone. A total of 50 metaphase cells exhibiting either single or double spots of hybridization signals were examined. Among them, 32 showed the specific signals on Chromosome 2q36. The genes for HOX4, fibronectin 1, villin 1, collagen type IV, Waardenburg syndrome type 1, alanine-glyoxylate aminotransferase, and glucagon are localized in the vicinity of the IRS-1 gene [34].

Hepatocytes are well known to be major target cells for insulin, together with muscles and adipose tissues. Insulin is also known to promote hepatocyte proliferation as a comitogenic factor. Sasaki et al. [34] reported an increase in content of tyrosine phosphorylated IRS-1 prior to stimulation of DNA synthesis during the course of liver regeneration induced by 2/3 hepatectomy, and PI-3 kinase was highly associated with IRS-1 following tyrosine phosphorylation in vivo [35]. We investigated the induction of ornithine decarboxylase (ODC) activity during liver regeneration after partial hepatectomy in IRS-1-deficient mice. Insulin induces ODC activity, a key enzyme of polyamine metabolism which is associated with cell proliferation [36]. No significant differences in ODC activity and time-related changes in ODC activity were observed between IRS-1-deficient mice and wild-type mice. Both groups also showed similar PI-3 kinase activity 1 h after partial hepatectomy [37]. Although these data show an apparent lack of importance of IRS-1 in hepatocyte proliferation, the results may arise as a result of the compensatory effects of IRS-2/pp190, a newly found second substrate of insulin receptor b-subunit [38]. The predicted amino acid sequences of IRS-1 and IRS-2 share approximately 70% homology in the N-terminal region and 35% in the C-terminal portion. IRS-2 has been reported to be expressed in various tissues under physiological conditions. The functional roles of these two IRSs are very similar with respect to the associations with PI-3 kinase and Grb-2. Thus, the IRSs may work as a multisite docking protein and play important roles in liver regeneration.

To investigate the expression and the subcellular localization of IRS-1 in hepatocytes, we obtained monoclonal antibodies by immunizing mice with a fusion protein containing the C-terminal portion of human IRS-1 (amino acids 778−1,243) and glutathione-S-transferase (GST). More than 30 hybridomas which produced immunoglobulin reacting with IRS-1 were isolated. Then seven MoAbs that were positive on Western blot analysis were further characterized and classified according to the pattern of recognition of the fusion protein used for immunization. These seven antibodies cross-react with rat, mouse and Chinese hamster IRS-1. All seven antibodies are of the IgG (k) subclass. On the basis of their reactivity to various portions of the GST-IRS-1 fusion protein construct, the epitopes for each antibody were estimated. One of the MoAbs, 6G5, recognizes a region located between amino acids 978−1,088 containing two possible tyrosine phosphorylation sites of IRS-1, which presumably are associated with PI-3 kinase. We have proved that 6G5 immunoprecipitates a 180 kDa tyrosine phosphoprotein corresponding to IRS-1 after insulin stimulation, and that it is an excellent MoAb for immunohistochemical studies using paraffin sections [39].

To further understand the contribution of IRS-1 in the development of liver diseases, we examined the expression of IRS-1 in various human liver diseases. Using an anti-IRS-1 monoclonal antibody, 6G5, immunohistochemical staining was performed on liver tissues from 11 patients with chronic hepatitis, 4 with liver cirrhosis and 18 with hepatocellular carcinoma. Serial sections from the same samples were also stained with anti-PCNA antibody to demonstrate DNA proliferation. In chronic hepatitis patients, IRS-1 staining was seen in the cytosol of hepatocytes. The intensity of the staining was parallel to the severity of chronic hepatitis. In cirrhotic patients, IRS-1 was strongly positive in regenerating nodules, and nuclei positively stained by anti-PCNA antibody were obvious in the same portion of the liver. In HCC patients, IRS-1 staining was stronger when HCC was highly differentiated. IRS-1 was expressed strongly in proliferating hepatocytes from patients with liver diseases, as shown in Table 5. These results suggest that IRS-1 may play an important part in transmitting the insulin signals to the intracellular regulators involved in liver diseases.

It is difficult to dissect the exact causes of insulin resistance-associated liver diseases, especially liver cirrhosis, presumably because multiple etiologies and genetic heterogeneity of hepatocytes in various liver diseases are likely to play a role in the respective conditions. Of the many proteins that are assumed to be involved in the action of insulin on the liver, mutation in insulin receptors and variations in number and affinity, substrates for insulin receptor kinase, post-

Table 5. Expression of IRS-1 in various human liver diseases.

Disease status	Age	Sex	Etiology	Differentiation	Anti-IRS-Mo Ab	Anti-PCNA Ab
CPH	39	M	HCV		1 +	2 +
	52	M	HCV		—	1 +
	24	F	HCV		—	1 +
CAH 2A	34	M	HCV		1 +	3 +
	49	F	HCV		1 +	1 +
	31	M	HCV		1 +	—
	27	M	HCV		1 +	2 +
	52	M	NBNC		1 +	3 +
CAH 2B	56	M	HCV		1 +	3 +
	24	F	HBV		2 +	3 +
	32	F	HCV		—	2 +
LC	61	M	HCV		2 +	4 +
	45	M	HCV		2 +	4 +
	62	M	HCV		2 +	3 +
	78	F	HCV		2 +	1 +
HCC	78	F	HCV	Well	1 +	2 +
	64	M	HCV	Well	1 +	1 +
	66	M	NBNC	Well	—	—
	53	M	HBV	Well	1 +	—
	48	M	HCV	Well	1 +	2 +
	66	M	HCV	Well	1 +	—
	63	F	HCV	Well	1 +	1 +
	62	M	HCV	Moderate	1 +	—
	61	M	HCV	Moderate	—	3 +
	63	F	HCV	Moderate	1 +	—
	61	F	HCV	Moderate	—	—
	74	M	HBV	Moderate	1 +	—
	67	M	HCV	Moderate	—	1 +
	64	M	HCV	Moderate	1 +	—
	56	M	HCV	Moderate	2 +	2 +
	50	F	HCV	Moderate	1 +	—
	58	F	HCV	Moderate	—	4 +
	54	M	HCV	Poorly	—	—

IRS-1 = insulin receptor substrate-1, CPH = chronic persistent hepatitis, CAH = chronic active hepatitis pathologically classified as CPH, CAH-2A and CAH-2B. LC = liver cirrhosis, HCC = hepatocellular carcinoma, HCV = hepatitis C virus, HBV = hepatitis B virus, NANB = non-A non-B hepatitis virus, M = male, F = female.

receptor signaling intermediates are possible candidates for causing insulin resistance in liver diseases. In this chapter, we can speculate that IRS-1 is one of the possible candidate proteins associated with hepatocyte functions including proliferation, and insulin resistance in liver diseases.

Conclusion

Hepatogenic diabetes is a distinctive disease condition manifested as carbohy-

98

drate intolerance in patients with decreased hepatic function, such as in cirrhosis. Carbohydrate intolerance associated with hyperinsulinemia and insulin resistance appears to be multifactorial in nature. The current thinking is that cirrhosis is associated with a combination of receptor binding and postbinding defects but the nature of the defects is not evident. It appears that the mechanisms of insulin resistance in cirrhosis and in primary diabetes mellitus are different. Therefore, hepatic diabetes should be differentiated from primary diabetes. It is important to stress that the carbohydrate intolerance in cirrhosis is rarely present as clinically significant hyperglycemia or necessitates treatment. Our studies described here show several distinctive differences between two diabetic states, including the effect on arteriosclerosis, galactose metabolism and prognosis. If a patient with cirrhosis has significant diabetes, one should probably consider this to represent the true entity of a systemic disease rather than a cause and effect relationship.

Acknowledgements

I am grateful to the staff of my Department, particularly to Akihiro Ohnishi MD, Akihiro Furusaka MD, Shigeto Murakami MD, Yasunori Kadowaki MD, Jun Hiramoto MD and Kazuo Nagayama MD for their helpful cooperation and to Miss Junko Hijikata for her secretarial work. I also greatly appreciate the contributions made by my colleagues Gohichiro Anan MD, Yutaka Kamio MD, Kimiharu Eto MD and Tomio Suda MD.

References

1. Naunyn B. Der Diabetes Mellitus. In: Nothnagel E (ed) Handbuch Spez Path Ther. Wien: A. Hoelder, 1906.
2. Taub SJ, Shlaes WH, Rice L. Liver dysfunction hyperglycemia: Its etiology and relation to diabetes mellitus. Ann Int Med 1945;22:852—862.
3. Leevy CM, Fineberg, JC, White TJ, Gnassi AM. Hyperglycemia and glycosuria in the chronic alcoholic with hepatic insufficiency. Clinical observations in 10 patients. Am J Med Sci 1952; 223:88—95.
4. Takahashi T, Fujisawa K, Tanaka T, Okabe K, Osamura H, Kurihara N, Nishikawa H, Kubo T, Ohkawa K, Kimura A. Whether is hepatogenic diabetes present or not? Nippon Rinsho 1967; 25:210—214. (In Japanese.)
5. Conn HO, Schreiber W, Elikington SG, Johnsin TR. Cirrhosis and Diabetes I. Increased incidence of diabetes in patients with Laennec's cirrhosis. Am J Dig Dis 1969;14:837—852.
6. Blei AT, Robbins DC, Drobny E, Baumann G, Rubenstein AH. Insulin resistence and insulin receptor in hepatic cirrhosis. Gastroenterology 1982;83:1191—1199.
7. Taylor R, Heine RJ, Collins J, James OF, Alberti KG. Insulin action in cirrhosis. Hepatology 1985;5:64—71.
8. Miyamoto I, Miyakoshi H, Nagai Y, Ohsawa K, Nishimura Y, Noto Y, Kobayashi K. Characterization of the insulin resistence in liver cirrhosis: a comparison with noninsulin dependent diabetes mellitus. Endocrinol Jpn 1992;39:421—429.
9. Oleffsky J, Lilly Lecture 1980: insulin resistance and insulin action. Diabetes 1980;30:148—162.
10. Anan G. Studies on hepatic injury and abnormal glucose tolerance test in the chronic liver dis-

eases. Jikeikai Med J 1976;91:1—15. (In Japanese.)

11. Kuzuya N, Abe M, Ueda H, Kuzuya K, Kosaka K, Goto Y, Shigeta Y, Baba Y, Hirata Y, Horiuchi H, Yamada K, Wada M. Report of the Committee on the Diagnostic Definition of Diabetes in Glucose Tolerance test. Jpn J Diabetic Soc 1970;13:1—7. (In Japanese.)

12. Seltzer HS, Allen EW et al. Insulin secretion in response to glycemic stimulus: relation of delayed initial release to carbohydrate intolerance in mild diabetes mellitus. J Clin Invest 1967; 46:323—335.

13. Sarles H. Chronic calcifying pancreatitis — chronic alcoholic pancreatitis. Gastroenterology 1974;66:604—616.

14. Spat SD, Rosenblatt P. The incidence of hypertension in portal cirrhosis: a study of 80 necropsied cases of portal cirrhosis. Ann Int Med 1949;31:479—483.

15. Loyke HF. The relationship of cirrhosis of the liver to hypertension: a study of 504 cases of cirrhosis of the liver. Am J Med 1955;230:627—632.

16. Creed DL, Baird WF, Fisher ER. The severity of aortic arteriosclerosis in certain disease: a necropsy study. Am J Med Sci 1955;230:385—391.

17. Osaka K, Ohno T, Harada M, Kawai B, Matsuo A, Inoue T, Ohnishi A, Tanaka T. Arteriosclerosis in liver cirrhosis. Kanzoh 1993;34:457—463. (In Japanese.)

18. Aiello LM, Cavallerano LD. Ocullar complication of diabetes mellitus. In: Losli's Diabetes Mellitus, 13th Ed. Philidelphia: Lea & Febiger, 1994;771—790.

19. The Diabetes Control and Complications Trial Research Group. The relationship of glycemic exposure (HbA1c) to the risk of development and progression of retinopathy in the Diabetes Control and Complication Trial. Diabetes 1995;44:968—983.

20. Engermann RL, Kern TS. Progression of incipient diabetic retinopathy during good glycemic control. Diabetes 1987;36:808—812.

21. Engermann RL, Kern TS. Experimental galactosemia produces diabetic-like retinopathy. Diabetes 1984;33:97—100.

22. Oltavi ZN, Milliman CL, Korsmeyer SJ. Bcl-2 heterodimerizes in vivo with a conserved homolog, Bax, that accelerates programmed cell death. Cell 1993;74:609—619.

23. Hayashi T, Yamaguchi H, Matsui K. Peroral galactose tolerance test. Jpn J Clin Pathol 1971; 19:10—13. (In Japanese.)

24. Shay H, Fieman P. The galactose tolerance test in jaundice; A consideration of the evidence permitting the measurement of galactose utilization by urinary excretion: Some sources error in its interpretation and an addition in routine technic. Ann Int Med 1937;10:1297—1303.

25. Eto K. Blood-glucose changes after oral galactose loads in chronic liver diseases. Jikeikai Med J 1982;29:263—274.

26. Ida T, Ozawa K, Honjo I. Glucose intolerance after massive liver resection in man and other mammals. Am J Surg 1975;129:523—527.

27. Ozawa K, Ida T, Yamada T, Honjo I. Significance of glucose tolerance as prognostic sign in hepatectomized patients. Am J Surg 1976;131:541—546.

28. Tanaka J, Ozawa K, Tobe T. Significancce of blood ketone body ratio as an indicator of hepatic cellular energy status in jaundiced rabbitts. Gastroenterology 1979;76:691—696.

29. Kamio Y. Changes of glucose tolerance and blood ketone bodies in liver cirrhotic patients after complication of hepatocellular carcinoma. Jikeikai Med J 1987;102:685—695. (In Japanese.)

30. White MF, Maron R, Kahn CR. Insulin rapidly stimulates tyrosine phosphorylation of a Mr-185,000 protein in intact cells. Nature 1985;318:183—185.

31. Nishiyama M, Wands J. Cloning and increased expression of an insulin receptor substrate-1 like gene in human hepatocellular carcinoma. Biochem Biophys Res Commun. 1992;183 280—285.

32. White M, Kahn CR. The insulin signaling system. J Biol Chem 1994;269:1—4.

33. Wang LM, Myers MG, Sun XJ, Aaronson SA, White M, Pierce JH. IRS-1: essential for insulin- and IL-4 stimulated mitogenesis in hematopoietic cells. Science, 1993;261(5128),1591—1594.

34. Sasaki Y, Zhang XF, Nisiyama M et al. Expression and phosphorylation of insulin receptor substrate-1 during rat liver regeneration. J Biol Chem 1993;268,3805—3808.

35. Pegg AE. Recent advances in the biochemistry of polyamines in eukaryotes. Biochem J 1986; 234:249—262.
36. Furusaka A, Nisiyama M, Tanaka T. Ornithine Decarboxylase Induction during liver Regeneration in IRS-1 Deficient Mice. Biochem Biophys Res Commun 1995;216:284—290.
37. Tobe K, Tamemoto H, Yamauchi T et al. Identification of a 190-kDa protein as a novel substrate for the insulin receptor kinase functionally similar to insulin receptor substrate-1. J Biol Chem 1995;270:5698—5701.
38. Nisiyama M, Furusaka A, Tanaka T et al. The human insulin receptor substrate-1 gene (IRS-1) is localized on 2q36. Genomics 1994;20:139—141.
39. Furusaka F, Nisiyama M, Tanaka T et al. Expression of insulin receptor substrate-1 in hepatocytes: an investigation using monoclonal antibodies. Cancer Lett 1994;84:85—92.

Progress in Hepatology, Volume 4.
Liver Cirrhosis Update.
M. Yamanaka et al., editors.

101

Nutritional treatment for abnormal lipid metabolism in cirrhotic patients

Misako Okita[1] and Akiharu Watanabe[2]

[1]*Department of Nutritional Science, Faculty of Health and Welfare Science, Okayama Prefectural University, Soja; and* [2]*The Third Department of Internal Medicine, Toyama Medical and Pharmaceutical University, Toyama, Japan*

Abstract. Patients with advanced liver cirrhosis showed low levels of phospholipid and cholesterol. Arachidonic acid in plasma phosphatidylcholine, phosphatidylinositol and phosphatidylethanolamine fractions was significantly decreased in cirrhotic patients. Significant decrease of eicosapentaenoic acid (EPA) and docosahexaenoic acid (DHA) in phospholipid was also observed. Some nutritional approaches for treatment of polyunsaturated fatty acid (PUFA) deficiency in cirrhotic patients were used in the present study. Dietary supplement of linoleic acid, EPA and DHA with 15 g of safflower oil and 80 g of fish resulted in elevation of linoleic acid and EPA of the plasma lipid, but failed to increase arachidonic acid. γ-Linolenic acid supplement using 10 g of evening primrose oil resulted in increased level of dihomo-γ-linolenic acid but not of arachidonic acid. These results indicate impaired delta-6 and delta-5 desaturase activity in the cirrhotic liver. Arachidonic acid-rich oil capsule administration was expected to improve arachidonic acid deficiency in the plasma phospholipid of cirrhotic patients. Because arachidonic acid is a very potent source of bioactive prostanoids, correction of arachidonic acid deficiency may play a beneficial role in the pathophysiology of liver cirrhosis.

Keywords: arachidonic acid, γ-linolenic acid, prostaglandin, phospholipid.

Introduction

Energy and protein malnutrition are commonly observed in patients with advanced liver cirrhosis, and many reports have focused on the nutritional treatment of protein malnutrition and of plasma amino acid imbalance using branched chain amino acid-supplemented nutritional products [1,2]. Although profound abnormalities in plasma-lipid profiles have been observed in liver cirrhotic patients [3], few attempts at normalizing the impaired lipid nutrition have been reported [4,5].

The liver plays a central role in lipid metabolism, as well as protein and other nutrient metabolisms. Its function includes intracellular lipid metabolism, such as β-oxidation, bile acid and lipid syntheses, and desaturation of fatty acids. Patients with advanced liver cirrhosis show low plasma levels of phospholipid, total cholesterol and cholesterol ester because of injured synthesis of these lipids in cirrhotic liver and low esterification of cholesterol. Plasma polyunsaturated

---

Address for correspondence: Misako Okita, Department of Nutritional Science, Faculty of Health and Welfare Science, Okayama Prefectural University, Soja 719-1112, Japan.

fatty acid (PUFA) deficiency is also commonly observed in patients with liver cirrhosis [3,6,7].

Some nutritional approaches for treatment of low plasma levels of PUFA in patients with liver cirrhosis are presented in the following pages.

Abnormal plasma lipid and fatty acid composition in cirrhotic patients

Plasma levels of total phospholipid, total cholesterol, cholesterol ester and triglyceride in patients with liver cirrhosis (16 males and 10 females, 50 ± 11 years of age, including patients with cirrhosis at the decompensated stage) are shown in Fig. 1. Plasma total phospholipid, total cholesterol and cholesterol ester levels were generally decreased in liver cirrhotic patients as the disease progressed. However, distribution of plasma triglyceride concentration was within normal range. The normal level of plasma triglyceride may be supported by the fact that the BMI (22.8 ± 0.6) in the cirrhotic patients did not show any decrease. Phospholipid and cholesterol, which are the principal components of all biomembranes, are both synthesized by the endoplasmic reticulum of many cells, particularly of the hepatocyte.

In plasma phospholipids, phosphatidylcholine is a prominent phospholipid, accounting for 80% of total phospholipids. In liver cirrhotic patients, as shown in Fig. 2, remarkable decreases in phosphatidylcholine, phosphatidylinositol and lysophosphatidylcholine were observed, but not in phosphatidylethanolamine. Phosphatidylcholine is responsible for the hydrophilic properties of the surface coat of lipoproteins. Phosphatidylethanolamine is converted to phosphatidylcho-

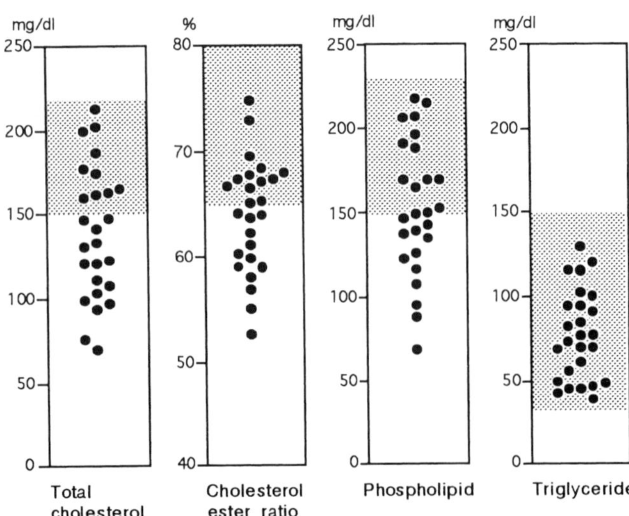

Fig. 1. Total cholesterol, phospholipid and triglyceride concentrations and cholesterol ester ratio in the plasma of cirrhotic patients. Shadows indicate the range observed in healthy controls.

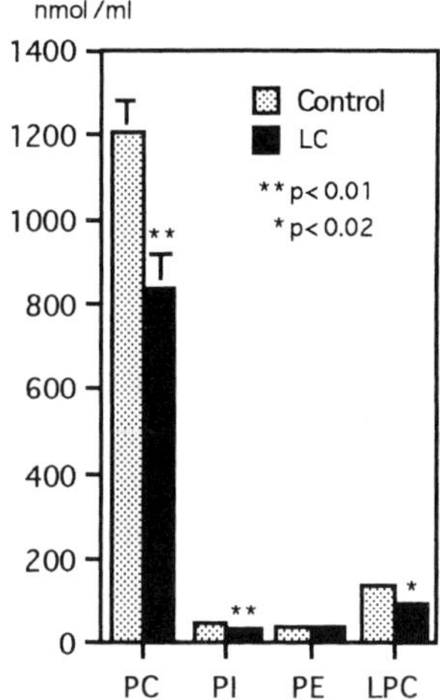

Fig. 2. Concentrations of each phospholipid fraction in the plasma of cirrhotic patients.

line by transmethylation of S-adenosylmethionine. It has been suggested that synthesis of S-adenosylmethionine is impaired in cirrhotic patients [8]. The limited transmethylation may be an explanation for the relatively high phosphatidylethanolamine levels in cirrhotic patients. Lysophosphatidylcholine is a normal constituent of human plasma and bound mostly to albumin and partly to various lipoproteins. Lysophosphatidylcholine can be generated from phosphatidylcholine by the action of plasma lecithin cholesterol acyltransferase (LCAT) or phospholipases. The low lysophosphatidylcholine levels appear to reflect low levels of phosphatidylcholine and albumin in the plasma of cirrhotic patients.

Plasma phospholipids are rich in PUFAs, and plasma cholesterol ester contains a very high level (more than 30% of total fatty acid) of linoleic acid. Therefore, a low plasma concentration of phospholipids and cholesterol esters contributes to the low plasma PUFA levels observed in cirrhotic patients (Fig. 3). Phosphatidyl-

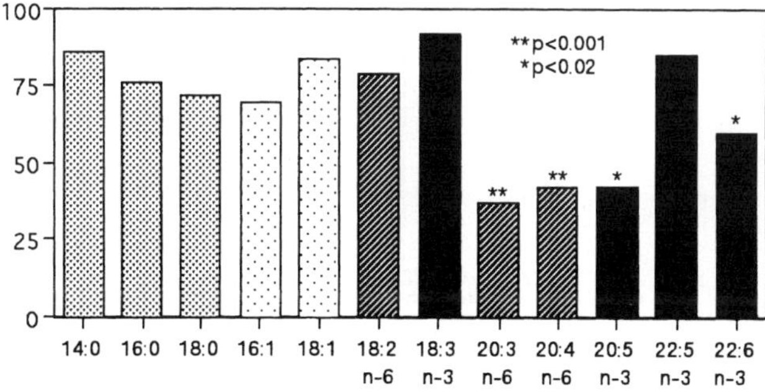

Fig. 3. Fatty acid composition in the plasma total lipids of cirrhotic patients. Each fatty acid concentration in the normal controls is expressed as 100.

ethanolamine is particularly rich in highly unsaturated fatty acids such as arachidonic acid (20:4n-6), eicosapentaenoic acid (EPA; 20:5n-3) and docosahexaenoic acid (DHA; 22:6n-3), and phosphatidylinositol contains high levels of arachidonic acid and DHA. In cirrhotic patients, significantly low levels of arachidonic acid in phosphatidylcholine, phosphatidylinositol and phosphatidylethanolamine were noted as shown in Fig. 4. Significantly low DHA levels were also noted in phosphatidylcholine and phosphatidylethanolamine. In contrast to arachidonic acid, linoleic acid (18:2n-6) did not decrease, and, in fact, it increased in phosphatidylinositol. Hence, arachidonic acid:linoleic acid molar ratios in phosphatidylinositol and phosphatidylethanolamine were significantly lower in cirrhotic patients than in normal subjects. The fatty acid composition of phospholipid contributes to the physical and biochemical properties of cell membranes and is influenced directly by the proportion of dietary PUFA.

Unsaturated fatty acids, linoleic acid and α-linolenic acid (18:3n-3), are essential for higher animals, since they are not synthesized in the body and must be supplied from the diet. Linoleic acid is converted to arachidonic acid via γ-linolenic acid (18:3n-6) and dihomo-γ-linolenic acid (20:3n-6), and α-linolenic acid is also converted to EPA and DHA by desaturation and chain elongation in the liver, as shown in Fig. 5. Impaired desaturation steps [6] may be a cause for deficiency of arachidonic acid and DHA in cirrhotic patients. A correlation between plasma PUFA concentration and the clinical data or the lipid intake in cirrhotic patients was observed in our previous study [9]. Arachidonic acid and DHA concentrations in the plasma total lipids correlated positively with KICG (r = 0.763, p < 0.05 and r = 0.771, p < 0.01, respectively) and serum albumin (r = 0.664, p < 0.05 and r = 0.779, p < 0.01) and negatively with the serum bilirubin

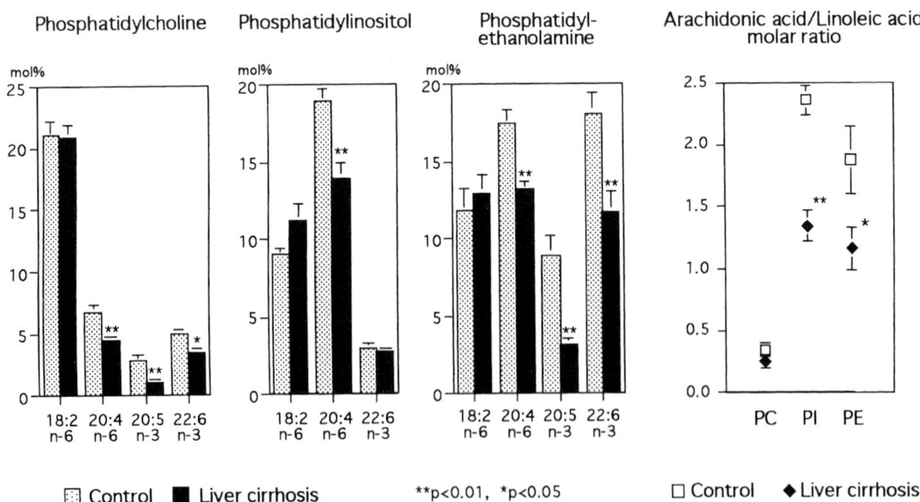

Fig. 4. Polyunsaturated fatty acid compositions and the arachidonic acid:linoleic acid molar ratios in the plasma phospholipids of cirrhotic patients.

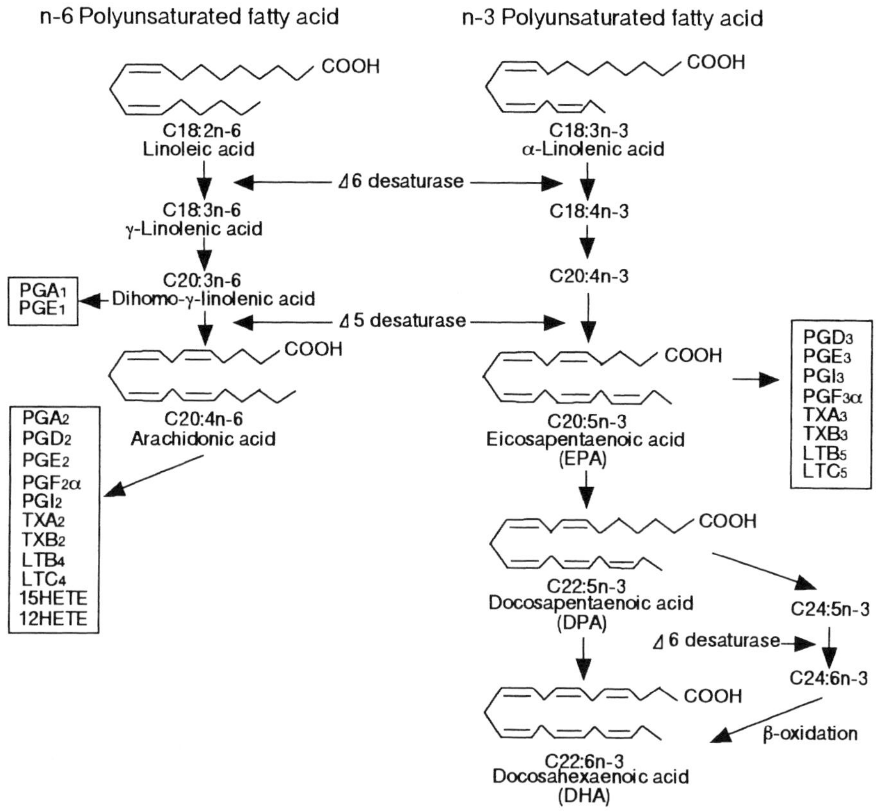

Fig. 5. Metabolic pathways for n-6 and n-3 polyunsaturated fatty acids.

level ($r = -0.693$, $p < 0.05$ and $r = -0.791$, $p < 0.01$). DHA concentrations in both lipid fractions correlated positively with the serum total cholesterol level. A significant negative correlation was observed between serum bilirubin level and arachidonic acid and DHA in the plasma total lipid fraction.

Most tissue has phospholipids in cell membranes, which are characterized by having predominantly PUFA, such as linoleic acid, arachidonic acid and EPA, esterified in position 2. On activation of phospholipase A2, arachidonic acid is normally released and oxidized by both lipoxygenase and cyclooxygenase. This action leads to the instantaneous biosynthesis of various prostagrandins, thromboxanes (TXs) or leukotriens of the 2-type. Dihomo-γ-linolenic acid and EPA are precursors of 1-type and 3-type prostanoids, i.e., PGE1 and PGE3, respectively. Prostanoids formed in the liver control several functions of hepatocytes, such as glycogenolysis [10,11] and DNA synthesis [12]. Pathogenesis of hepatorenal syndrome [13], platelet dysfunction [14], and ascites retention [15], which are frequently observed in liver cirrhosis, are also suggested to be related to prostanoid formation. An increased urinary excretion of 6-keto PGF1α which is a stable metabolite of prostacyclin (PGI2), in cirrhotic patients [16] and an elevated level of plasma 6-keto PGF1α in cirrhotic rats induced by CCl4 [17,18] have been reported. Although the mechanism is not clear, enhanced synthesis of prostaglandins may be postulated as a possible cause of decreased arachidonic acid content in plasma phospholipids.

Cell membrane function depends primarily on the fluidity of the lipid matrix of the cell. PUFA content is thought to play a major role in cell membrane fluidity and integrity [19]. Changes in membrane fluidity in both hepatocyte membranes [20] and erythrocyte membranes [21] have been reported in liver disease.

Multivariate analysis revealed a relationship between plasma PUFA deficiency and survival in advanced cirrhosis of the liver [22]. Therefore, it is expected that dietary treatment of PUFA deficiency may prevent the impairments of the function of various organs in liver cirrhosis.

Inadequate dietary intake of PUFA in cirrhotic patients

A low intake of dietary fat is suspected as a reason for the decrease in plasma PUFAs [7]. Primary bile acids are produced in the liver and conjugated with glycine and taurine. These conjugated acids are extremely active in the formation of micelles, which enhance the enzymatic hydrolysis of dietary triglyceride to monoglyceride and fatty acid, and promote absorption of the end products of lipolysis. Low dietary fat intake, therefore, has been recommended in patients with reduced biliary secretion because of serious liver disease such as acute hepatitis and decompensated liver cirrhosis. However, it has been reported that forced feeding with a high-energy, high-protein and high-fat diet could be tolerated well in patients with acute viral hepatitis [23].

As has been mentioned, two PUFAs, linoleic and α-linolenic acid, are known to be essential for higher animals, including man. Therefore, these animals depend on dietary fat, mainly vegetable oil, to meet these essential fatty acid requirements. In humans, the dietary requirement for linoleic acid may be 5–10% of total energy, and 0.5–1.0% of total energy for α-linolenic acid [24]. In our earlier study [8], the cirrhotic patients consumed only 6.3 g linoleic acid per day (3% of total energy) and 0.36% of energy of α-linolenic acid from their diet. It was reported that conversions of α-linolenic acid to n-3 fatty acid metabolites and linoleic acid to n-6 fatty acid metabolites in normal humans were 11–18.5% and 1.0–2.2%, respectively [25]. A low intake of essential fatty acids over a long period may induce a deficiency not only of linoleic acid and α-linolenic acid but also of their metabolites. Continued feeding of an essential fatty-acid-deficient diet leads to partial replacement of arachidonic acid by eicosatrienoic acid (20:3n-9), which is a substrate for lipoxygenase but not for cycrooxygenase. Additionally, a low intake of fish rich in EPA and DHA might induce low levels of plasma EPA and DHA.

Dietary treatment of PUFA deficiency in cirrhotic patients

Fish and safflower oil supplement

Vegetable oils, particularly safflower oil, contain a high level of linoleic acid, and several fish, such as sardine, mackerel and tuna, are rich in highly unsaturated n-3 fatty acid, EPA, docosapentaenoic acid (DPA; 22:5n-3) and DHA. Nine decompensated cirrhotic patients (four males and five females, 47 ± 12 years of age) were served a PUFA-supplemented diet containing 80 g of fish rich in EPA and DHA and 15 g of safflower oil (76.4% linoleic acid) per day for 2 weeks [9]. Safflower oil was incorporated into mayonnaise or salad dressings. All the cirrhotic patients received a special hospital diet for liver disease (standard liver diet) for at least 7 days prior to the experimental diet. Two diets, standard liver diet and PUFA-supplemented diet, were isocaloric (2,000 kcal/day) and isoprotein (70 g/day). Dietary fat and PUFA intake from the two different diets are presented in Table 1. The changes in plasma fatty acid composition in total lipid fractions following the PUFA-supplemented diet are shown in Fig. 6. A significant increase in plasma linoleic acid and EPA concentrations was recognized following the PUFA-supplemented diet. However, only a small, insignificant increase was observed in dihomo-γ-linolenic acid and arachidonic acid, which are metabolites of linoleic acid, and also in DHA. Supplementation of a large quantity of PUFA may be needed to obtain a significant increase in plasma arachidonic acid and DHA in cirrhotic patients having impaired synthesis of these fatty acids.

Evening primrose oil-supplemented diet

Evening primrose oil is a naturally occurring plant oil containing γ-linolenic acid. γ-Linolenic acid is the first metabolite produced by delta-6 desaturase in the pathway from linoleic acid to arachidonic acid. Delta-6 desaturase is a rate-limiting step in the conversion of both linoleic and α-linolenic acid. γ-Linolenic acid supplement, therefore, was expected to increase dihomo-γ-linolenic and arachidonic acids.

Table 1. Dietary intake of fat and PUFAs in decompensated cirrhotic patients.

	Standard liver diet	PUFA-supplemented diet
Total fat (g/day)	30 ± 10	42 ± 12[a]
Fatty acid (g/day)		
Linoleic acid	6.3 ± 2.0	13.9 ± 2.5[b]
α-Linolenic acid	0.6 ± 0.2	0.8 ± 0.6
Arachidonic acid	0.10 ± 0.06	0.12 ± 0.06
Eicosapentaenoic acid	0.11 ± 0.08	0.30 ± 0.17[b]
Docosahexaenoic acid	0.16 ± 0.10	0.41 ± 0.20[b]

Values are given as mean ± SD; [a]p < 0.05; [b]p < 0.01

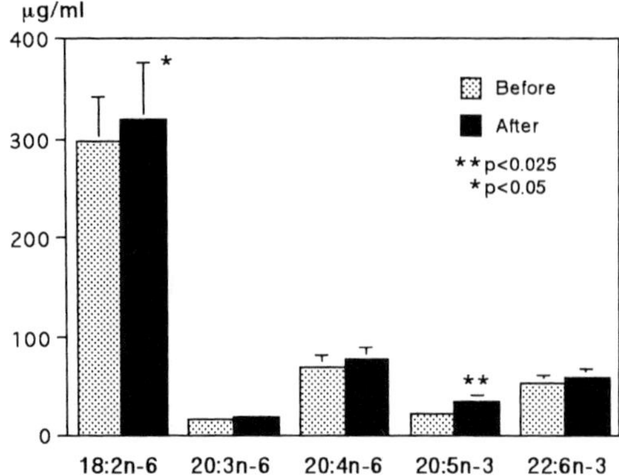

Fig. 6. The changes in plasma fatty acid composition in total lipid fractions of cirrhotic patients following fish- and safflower-oil-supplemented diet.

Seven decompensated cirrhotic patients (five males and two females, 57 ± 8 years of age) were served 10 g of evening primrose oil (68% linoleic acid and 9% γ-linolenic acid) incorporated into mayonnaise daily for 2 weeks. The changes in plasma PUFA following the evening primrose oil-supplemented diet are shown in Fig. 7. The relative compositions of linoleic acid, γ-linolenic acid and dihomo-γ-linolenic acid in plasma total lipid fraction increased significantly, but only a small, insignificant increase was observed in plasma arachidonic acid. These data may suggest that not only delta-6, but also delta-5 desaturase in the conversion pathway of linoleic acid and α-linolenic acid are impaired in the cirrhotic liver and, hence, arachidonic acid formation may be retained.

Although arachidonic acid was not significantly increased, bleeding time was shortened from 4.6 ± 0.5 min to 2.9 ± 1.0 min (p < 0.05) following the evening

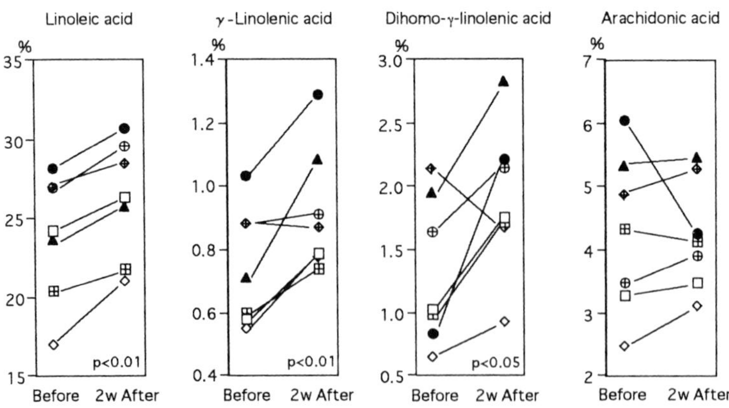

Fig. 7. The changes in plasma polyunsaturated fatty acid following evening primrose-oil-supplemented diet in cirrhotic patients.

primrose oil-supplemented diet. Cyclooxygenase converts arachidonic acid via several intermediates into TXA2, which induces platelet aggregation. The formation of TXA2 by blood platelets may be influenced by γ-linolenic acid supplement using evening primrose oil.

Administration of arachidonic acid-rich oil capsules

Dietary treatment of cirrhotic patients with safflower oil or evening primrose oil did not have a significant effect on plasma arachidonic acid deficiency. Therefore, oral administration of arachidonic acid-rich oil was tested in cirrhotic patients, and the changes in fatty acid composition in plasma phospholipid were evaluated [26].

Arachidonic acid-rich triglyceride manufactured and purified from Mortierella alpina S-4 strain (Suntory, Tokyo, Japan) was used together with EPA- and DHA-rich fish oils. The three kinds of oil were mixed and wrapped in soft capsules. The selected fatty acid composition of the soft oil capsules is shown in Table 2. Twelve capsules containing 421 mg arachidonic acid, 271 mg EPA and 408 mg DHA were administered to three cirrhotic patients (two males and one female, 68 ± 6 years of age) and three controls (males, 51 ± 16 years of age) in the early morning. The subjects skipped breakfast and received a very low-fat diet for lunch (443 kcal, 9.1 g protein and 0.1 g fat) and supper (402 kcal, 11.6 g protein and 0.1 g fat).

Before the administration of arachidonic acid-rich oil capsules, dihomo-γ-linolenic acid, arachidonic acid and EPA levels in serum total lipid and phospholipid were significantly lower in cirrhotic patients than in control subjects (Table 3). The arachidonic acid:linoleic acid molar ratio of serum total lipid was also significantly lower in cirrhotic patients than in controls. After the administration of arachidonic acid-rich oil capsules, arachidonic acid increased in the serum phospholipid. The arachidonic acid:linoleic acid molar ratio of phospholipid in

Table 2. Fatty acid composition of arachidonic acid-rich oil capsules.

	mg%
Myristic acid (14:0)	12.5
Palmitic acid (16:0)	18.5
Palmitoleic acid (16:1n-7)	4.2
Stearic acid (18:0)	5.8
Oleic acid (18:1n-9)	18.9
Linoleic acid (18:2n-6)	8.8
α-Linolenic acid (18:3n-6)	1.4
γ-Linolenic acid (18:3n-3)	0.3
Dihomo-γ-linolenic acid (20:3n-6)	2.0
Arachidonic acid (20:4n-6)	14.0
Eicosapentaenoic acid (20:5n-3)	9.0
Docosahexaenoic acid (22:6n-3)	13.6

110

Table 3. Fatty acid concentrations of the serum phospholipid in cirrhotic patients and control subjects before and 24 h after arachidonic acid-rich oil capsule administration.

	Control subjects		Cirrhotic patients	
	Before	24 h after	Before	24 h after
Linoleic acid	54.5 ± 2.3	49.9 ± 12.0	48.8 ± 29.9	39.6 ± 19.4
Dihomo-γ-linolenic acid	10.8 ± 2.1	12.9 ± 2.7	4.8 ± 0.9[a]	5.1 ± 1.3
Arachidonic acid	26.7 ± 6.5	41.2 ± 10.0[b]	17.3 ± 1.9[a]	21.5 ± 7.5[b]
EPA	5.3 ± 1.3	5.2 ± 2.2	2.5 ± 0.4[a]	2.9 ± 0.9
DHA	21.0 ± 10.1	25.8 ± 10.3	12.3 ± 0.8	12.5 ± 2.0
Arachidonic acid:linoleic acid molar ratio	0.50 ± 0.18	0.80 ± 0.25[b]	0.46 ± 0.29	0.72 ± 0.35[b]

Values are in µmol/100 ml and expressed as mean ± SD; [a]$p < 0.05$ for comparison of control subjects with cirrhotic patients; [b]$p < 0.05$ for comparison of before and 24 h after. Wilcoxon's signed-ranks test.

cirrhotic patients elevated to the same degree as in control subjects after arachidonic acid-rich oil capsule administration. Arachidonic acid, EPA and DHA molar percentages in serum phospholipid before and 24 h after administration of arachidonic acid-rich oil capsules are illustrated in Fig. 8. Only a slight increase was observed in EPA and DHA concentrations in phospholipid 24 h after arachidonic acid-rich oil capsules containing EPA- and DHA-rich fish oil administration to cirrhotic patients. These results suggest that arachidonic acid supplemented by arachidonic acid-rich oil with fish oil corrected the deficiency of arachidonic acid, but a longer period of supplementation is needed to evaluate the usefulness of arachidonic acid supplementation in decompensated cirrhotic patients.

Our previous study of ethanol-treated rats fed with lard [27] revealed that large amounts of arachidonic acid (ethyl ester form, 3% of diet by weight) lowered se-

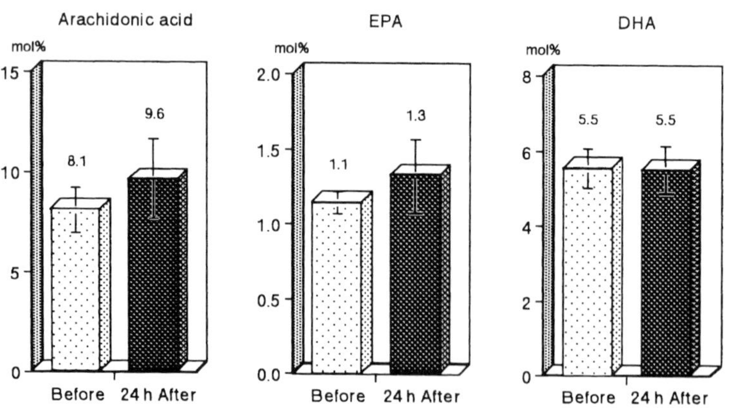

Fig. 8. The arachidonic acid, EPA and DHA molar percentages in serum phospholipids of cirrhotic patients before and 24 h after the administration of arachidonic acid-rich oil capsules.

rum ALT activity and liver triglyceride content and increased liver 6-keto-PGF1α. From the animal study, arachidonic acid supplement was expected to protect against liver injury induced by ethanol.

Arachidonic acid is considered a harmful substance if it is consumed in large amounts. However, a human dietary arachidonic acid supplement study, reported recently by Nelson et al. [28] revealed that dietary arachidonic acid had no deleterious effect on platelet aggregation [29] and plasma lipids [30]. In Nelson et al.'s study, a triglyceride produced by algae that contained 50% arachidonic acid (1.5 g arachidonic acid/day) was fed to healthy male (nonobese) subjects for 50 days. Plasma phospholipid and cholesterol ester in the study showed a marked increase in their content of arachidonic acid. A remarkable increase in the excretion of 11-dehydrothromboxan B2, a metabolite of TX, and 6-keto-PGF1α was observed after the high arachidonic acid diet [31].

Since EPA and DHA have a greater affinity for the position 2 of biomembrane phospholipids, a large intake of EPA and DHA causes a reduction of arachidonic acid levels in phospholipid. What is the best composition of dietary fatty acid? How much arachidonic acid should be supplemented for sufficient production of prostaglandins protecting against liver injury? Further clinical trials should be conducted to answer these questions.

Several natural or microbiologically obtained oils are now available commercially. Table 4 provides a list of edible oils important for nutritional management of diseases. The rationale and status of both n-3 and n-6 fatty acid dietary supplement in patients with inflammatory disease have been reviewed by Kremer [32]. Borage oil is richer in γ-linolenic acid than evening primrose oil. In a hamster model for bleomycin-induced lung fibrosis, γ-linolenic acid seemed to attenuate inflammation and fibrosis [33]. Flaxseed, rapeseed and perillaseed oils contain high levels of α-linolenic acid, and flaxseed has been used for the treatment of autoimmune disease [34], and dietary fish-oil-reduced hyperlipidemia in hepatoma-bearing rats [35].

Table 4. Selected triglyceride fatty acid composition of important edible oils.

	Fatty acid (weight %)								
	16:0	18:0	18:1 n-9	18:2 n-6	18:3 n-6	20:4 n-6	18:3 n-3	20:5 n-3	22:6 n-3
Olive oil	9.9	3.2	75.0	10.4	—	—	0.8	—	—
Safflower oil	7.3	2.6	13.4	76.4	—	—	0.2	—	—
Evening primrose oil	6.8	1.5	9.3	72.3	8.8	—	—	—	—
Borage oil	10.6	3.6	16.0	40.2	22.8	—	—	—	—
GLARO25	15.3	1.2	38.3	14.5	25.3	—	—	—	—
SUN-TGA25	13.5	6.1	13.2	23.5	1.9	24.6	1.8	—	—
Rapeseed oil	4.0	1.7	58.6	21.8	—	—	10.8	—	—
Perilla oil	7.0	2.2	28.7	14.9	—	—	45.5	—	—
Fish oil (EPA rich)	6.9	0.3	10.5	—	—	2.9	0.1	28.3	14.5
Fish oil (DHA rich)	16.5	3.5	18.3	1.4	—	—	—	6.2	28.0

112

Conclusions

Arachidonic acid deficiency may contribute to the impairment of the function of various organs in liver cirrhosis. Because arachidonic acid is a very potent source of bioactive prostanoids, arachidonic acid deficiency plays a large role in the pathophysiology of liver cirrhosis. Nutritional treatment using special oil containing not only n-6, but also n-3 PUFA seems to be necessary to maintain normal composition of plasma fatty acid and to protect against various complications observed in liver cirrhosis.

References

1. Fischer JE, Rosen HM, Ebeid AM, James JH, Keane JM, Soeters PB. The effect of normalization of plasma amino acids on hepatic encephalopathy in man. Surgery 1976;80:77—91.
2. Okita M, Watanabe A, Nagashima H. Nutritional treatment of liver cirrhosis by branched-chain amino acid-enriched nutrient mixture. J Nutr Sci Vitaminol 1985;31:291—303.
3. Johnson SB, Gordon E, McClain C, Low G, Holman RT. Abnormal polyunsaturated fatty acid patterns of serum lipids in alcoholism and cirrhosis: arachidonic acid deficiency in cirrhosis. Proc Natl Acad Sci USA 1985;82:1815—1818.
4. Rimola A, Ginés P, Cusó E, Camps J, Gaya J, Arroyo V, Rodés J. Prostaglandin precursor fatty acids in cirrhosis with ascites: Effect of linoleic acid infusion in functional renal failure. Clin Sci 1988;74:613—619.
5. Das UN, Sahay BK, Kumar S, Rao MH. Beneficial effect of essential fatty acids in cirrhosis of the liver. J API 1987;35:139—140.
6. Cabré E, Periago JL, Abad-Lacruz A, González-Huix F, González J, Esteve-Comas M, Fernández-Bañares F, Planas R, Gil A, Sánchez-Medina F, Gassull MA. Plasma fatty acid profile in advanced cirrhosis: unsaturation deficit of lipid fractions. Am J Gastroenterol 1990;85: 1597—1604.
7. Okita M, Watanabe A, Tsuji T. Lipid malnutrition of patients with liver cirrhosis: effect of low intake of dietary lipid on plasma fatty acid composition. Acta Med Okayama 1989;43:39—45.
8. Horowitz JH, Rypins EB, Henderson JM, Heymsfield SB, Moffitt SD, Bain RP, Chawla RK, Bleier JC, Rudman D. Evidence for impairment of transsulfuration pathway in cirrhosis. Gastroenterol 1981;81:668—675.
9. Okita M, Watanabe A, Tsuji T. Beneficial effect of polyunsaturated fatty acid-supplemented diet on altered composition of plasma fatty acids in patients with liver cirrhosis. J Clin Biochem Nutr 1989;6:213—220.
10. Brass EP, Garrity MJ. Effect of E-series prostaglandins on cyclic AMP-dependent and -independent hormone-stimulated glycogenolysis in hepatocytes. Diabetes 1985;34:291—294.
11. Okumura T, Sago T, Saito K. Effect of prostaglandins and their analogues on hormone-stimulated glycogenolysis in primary cultures of rat hepatocytes. Biochem Biophys Acta 1988;958: 179—187.
12. Andreis PG, Whitfield JF, Armato U. Stimulation of DNA synthesis and mitosis of hepatocytes in primary cultures of neonatal rat liver by arachidonic acid prostaglandins. Exp Cell Res 1981;134:265—272.
13. Gentilini P. Cirrhosis, renal function and NSAIDs. J Hepatology 1993;19:200—203.
14. Laffi G, La Villa G, Pinzani M, Ciabattoni G, Patrignani P, Mannelli M, Comimelli F, Gentilini P. Altered renal and platelet arachidonic acid metabolism in cirrhosis. Gastroenterol 1986;90: 274—282.
15. Zipser RD, Radvan GH, Kronborg IJ, Duke R, Little TE. Urinary thromboxane B2 and prostaglandin E2 in the hepatorenal syndrome: evidence for increased vasoconstrictor and decreased

vasodilator factors. Gastroenterol 1983;84:697—703.

16. Guarner C, Soriano G, Such J, Teixido M, Ramis I, Bulbena O, Rosello J, Guarner F, Gelpi E, Balanzo J, Vilardell F. Systemic prostacyclin in cirrhotic patients. Gastroenterol 1992;102: 303—309.

17. Oberti F, Sogni P, Cailmail S, Moreau R, Pipy B, Lebree D. Role of prostacyclin in hemodynamic alterations in conscious rats with extrahepatic or intrahepatic portal hypertension. Hepatology 1993;18:621—627.

18. Sitzmann JV, Cambell K, Wu Y, St.Clair C. Prostacyclin production in acute, chronic, and long-term experimental portal hypertension. Surgery 1994;115:290—294.

19. Kakimoto H, Imai Y, Kawata S, Inada M, Ito T, Matsuzawa Y. Altered lipid composition and differential changes in activities of membrane-bound enzymes of erythrocytes in hepatic cirrhosis. Metabolism 1995;44:825—832.

20. Schüller A, Solís-Herruzo JA, Moscat J, Fernandez-Checa JC, Municio AM. The fluidity of liver plasma membranes from patients with different types of liver injury. Hepatology 1986;6: 714—717.

21. Owen JS, Bruckdorfer R, Day RC, Day RC, McIntyre N. Decreased erythrocyte membrane fluidity and altered lipid composition in human liver disease. J Lipid Res 1982;23:124—132.

22. Cabré E, Abad-Lacruz A, Núñez MC, González-Huix F, Frenández-Bañares F, Gl A, Esteve-Comas M, Moreno J, Planas R, Guilera M, Gassull MA. The relationship of plasma polyunsaturated fatty acid deficiency with survival in advanced liver cirrhosis. Multivar Anal 1993;88: 718—722.

23. Chalmers TC, Eckhardt RD, Reynolds WE, Cigarroa JG, Deane N, Reifenstein RW, Smith CW, Davidson CS. The treatment of acute infectious hepatitis. Controlled studies of the effects of diet, rest, and physical reconditioning on the acute course of the disease and on the incidence of relapses and residual abnormalities. J Clin Invest 1955;34:1163—1235.

24. Linscheer WG, Vergroesen AJ. Lipids. In: Shils ME, Olson JA, Shike M (eds) Modern Nutrition in Health and Disease, vol 2. Philadelphia: Lea & Febiger, 1994;47—88.

25. Emken EA, Adlof RO, Gulley M. Dietary linoleic acid influences desaturation and acylation of deuterium-labeled linoleic and linolenic acids in young adult males. Biochem Biophys Acta 1994;1213:277—288.

26. Okita M, Miyamoto A, Wakabayashi H, Watanabe A. Improvement of polyunsaturated fatty acid deficiency in decompensated cirrhotic patients by arachidonic acid-rich oil capsules. In: Yasugi T, Nakamura H, Soma M (eds) Advances in Polyunsaturated Fatty Acid Research. North-Holland: Elsevier 1993;241—242.

27. Okita M, Suzuki K, Sasagawa T, Yamamoto J, Miyamoto A, Wakabayashi H, Watanabe A. Effect of arachidonate on lipid metabolism in ethanol-treated rats fed with lard. J Nutr Sci Vitaminol 1997;43:311—326.

28. Nelson GJ, Kelly DS, Emken EA, Phonney SD, Kyle D, Ferretti A. A human dietary arachidonic acid supplementation study conducted in a metabolic research unit: rationale and design. Lipids 1997;32:415—420.

29. Nelson GJ, Schmidt PC, Bartolini G, Kelley DS, Kyle D. The effect of dietary arachidonic acid on platelet function, platelet fatty acid composition, and blood coagulation in humans. Lipids 1997;32:421—425.

30. Nelson GJ, Schmidt PC, Bartolini G, Kelley DS, Phinney SD, Kyle D, Silbermann S, Schaefer EJ. The effect of dietary arachidonic acid on plasma lipoprotein distributions, apoproteins, blood lipid levels, and tissue fatty acid composition in humans. Lipids 1997;32:427—433.

31. Ferretti A, Nelson GJ, Schmidt PC, Kelley DS, Bartolini G, Flangan VP. Increased dietary arachidonic acid enhances the synthesis of vasoactive eicosanoids in humans. Lipids 1997;32: 435—439.

32. Kremer JM. Effects of modulation of inflammatory and immune parameters in patients with rheumatic and inflammatory disease receiving dietary supplementation of n-3 and n-6 fatty acids. Lipids 1996;31:S243—S247.

33. Ziboh VA, Yun M, Hyde DM, Giri SN. γ-Linolenic acid-containing diet attenuates bleomycin-induced lung fibrosis in hamsters. Lipids 1997;32:759—767.
34. Clark WF, Parbtani A, Huff MW, Spanner E, de Salis H, Chin-Yee I, Philbrick DJ, Holub BJ. Flaxseed: a potential treatment for lupus nephritis. Kidney Int 1995;48:475—480.
35. Kawasaki M, Yagasaki K, Miura Y, Funabiki R. Reduction of hyperlipidemia in hepatoma-bearing rats by dietary fish oil. Lipids 1995;30:431—436.

Energy metabolism determines the survival of patients with liver cirrhosis

Masahiro Tajika, Masahiko Kato, Yoshiyuki Miwa, Hiromi Mohri and Hisataka Moriwaki

First Department of Internal Medicine, Gifu University School of Medicine, Gifu, Japan

Abstract. Patients with liver cirrhosis have protein-energy malnutrition. We characterized the energy metabolism and analyzed its effect on survival in cirrhotics. Ninety-eight patients and 20 healthy controls received indirect calorimetry after an overnight bed rest and a fast. Resting energy expenditure and nonprotein respiratory quotient were measured. Survival of cirrhotics was followed up thereafter for 7 years. Increase in resting energy expenditure and decrease in nonprotein respiratory quotient were significant in liver cirrhosis when compared with controls ($p < 0.01$, $p < 0.001$, respectively). Survival rate estimated by the Kaplan-Meier method was significantly lower in patients with low nonprotein respiratory quotient (< 0.85) than those with the value above 0.85 ($p < 0.05$). The proportional hazards model demonstrated that serum albumin (relative risk, 0.195, 95% confidence interval, 0.073–0.523), nonprotein respiratory quotient (0.000, 0.000–0.023) and resting energy expenditure (0.007, 0.000–0.531) were independent significant factors to determine the survival of cirrhotics. Nonprotein respiratory quotient significantly correlated with parameters of functional reserve of the liver such as serum albumin. Resting energy expenditure significantly correlated with blood ammonia and anthropometrical parameters including body mass index. Energy metabolism determines the survival of patients with liver cirrhosis. Further investigations are required to elucidate if nutritional support for energy malnutrition improves the prognosis in cirrhotics.

Keywords: indirect calorimetry, nonprotein respiratory quotient, resting energy expenditure.

Introduction

Patients with liver cirrhosis have protein-energy malnutrition [1]. It is established that protein nutritional state determines the survival of cirrhotic patients [2]. Nutritional support using branched-chain amino acids for protein malnutrition improves the prognosis of these patients in part [3] although there are some criticisms of such a therapeutic strategy [4,5]. Recent studies revealed that energy nutritional state also determines the prognosis of alcoholic liver cirrhosis [6—9] and, furthermore, survival after liver transplantation in cirrhotics [10]. However, only limited information is currently available as to the energy nutritional state of the patients with viral liver cirrhosis. We characterized the energy metabolism and analyzed its possible effect on survival in a population of cirrhotic patients which mainly consisted of chronic hepatitis virus infection.

Address for correspondence: Hisataka Moriwaki MD, PhD, Professor, First Department of Internal Medicine, Gifu University School of Medicine, 40 Tsukasa-Machi, Gifu 500, Japan. Tel.: +81-58-267-2843. Fax: +81-58-262-8484. E-mail: hmori@cc.gifu-u.ac.jp

Characteristics of energy metabolism in liver cirrhosis

Energy metabolism was analyzed using indirect calorimetry in a similar manner to previous reports [11] in 98 patients and 20 controls. Clinical and biochemical characteristics of the subjects are given in Table 1. Etiologies of liver cirrhosis were hepatitis B virus in 10 patients, hepatitis C virus in 66, both hepatitis B and C viruses positive in one, non-B non-C virus in six, alcohol in 13 and primary biliary cirrhosis in two.

Indirect calorimetry was performed for 30 min after an overnight bed rest and a fast. In the preceding days before calorimetry, all subjects ate in full a standard diet containing a total energy of 33 kcal/kg/day, 1.3 g protein/kg/day, and 0.6 g fat/kg/day (energy ratio 16%).

Measured parameters by calorimetry were oxygen consumption per minute (VO_2) and carbon dioxide production per minute (VCO_2). Urine samples were collected for 24 h before and during calorimetry, and urinary nitrogen concentration was determined by the pyrochemiluminescence method [12]. Resting energy expenditure (REE), nonprotein respiratory quotient (npRQ) and oxidation volumes of carbohydrate (CHO), fat (FAT) and protein (PRO) were estimated by the following equations [11]:

$$\text{REE (kcal/day)} = 3.82VO_2 + 1.22VCO_2 - 1.99UN$$
$$\text{npRQ} = (VCO_2 - 4.89UN)/(VO_2 - 6.04UN)$$
$$\text{CHO (g/day)} = 4.12VCO_2 - 2.91VO_2 - 2.54UN$$
$$\text{FAT (g/day)} = 1.69VO_2 - 1.69VCO_2 - 1.94UN$$
$$\text{PRO (g/day)} = 6.25UN$$

Table 1. Clinical and biochemical profiles of controls and patients with liver cirrhosis.

	Controls (n = 20)	Liver cirrhosis (n = 98)
Age (years)	52 ± 15	60 ± 9[a]
Gender (M/F)	12/8	52/46
Total protein (g/dl)	7.3 ± 0.5	7.1 ± 0.8
Albumin (g/dl)	4.3 ± 0.6	3.0 ± 0.6[b]
Total bilirubin (mg/dl)	0.8 ± 0.1	1.9 ± 1.8[b]
AST (IU/l)	21 ± 4	64 ± 25[b]
ALT (IU/l)	23 ± 7	48 ± 26[b]
Hepaplastin test (%)	92 ± 8	58 ± 24[b]
Blood urea nitrogen (mg/dl)	14.2 ± 3.0	14.8 ± 7.3
Creatinine (mg/dl)	1.0 ± 0.2	0.9 ± 0.4
Urinary urea nitrogen (g/day)	7.4 ± 2.8	6.6 ± 2.8
Fasting blood glucose (mg/dl)	92 ± 2	116 ± 43[b]
Total cholesterol (mg/dl)	196 ± 35	116 ± 37[b]
Triglyceride (mg/dl)	103 ± 62	73 ± 35[a]
Fischer's ratio	3.5 ± 0.4	1.6 ± 0.7[b]

Values are expressed as mean ± SD. [a]$p < 0.05$; [b]$p < 0.001$ as compared to controls. AST: aspartate aminotransferase; ALT: alanine aminotransferase.

where UN indicates the estimated urinary excretion of nitrogen per day. REE was standardized by the basal metabolic rate calculated by the Harris-Benedict formula [13] to avoid the possible effects of age, gender, height and body weight [14]:

REE/BMR = estimated REE/calculated BMR

Oxidation rates of carbohydrates (%CHO), fat (%FAT) and protein (%PRO) were expressed as a percentage of total generated energy:

%CHO (or %FAT, %PRO) = 4.18CHO (or 9.46FAT, 4.32PRO) × 100 / (4.18CHO + 9.46FAT + 4.32PRO)

An increase in resting energy expenditure and a decrease in nonprotein respiratory quotient were significant in liver cirrhosis when compared with controls ($p < 0.01$, $p < 0.001$, respectively) (Fig. 1). A decrease in nonprotein respiratory quotient was brought about by significantly lower oxidation rate of carbohydrate and higher oxidation rate of fat in liver cirrhosis than those in controls ($p < 0.001$, $p < 0.001$, respectively) (Fig. 2). Changes in oxidation rates of nutrients as described above significantly correlated with the progression of disease severity of liver cirrhosis defined by the modified Child's classification (Fig. 3). Subsequently, nonprotein respiratory quotient also significantly correlated with the disease severity of cirrhotics (Fig. 4). We then defined the normal energy nutritional state as those who have resting energy expenditure and nonprotein respiratory quotient within the mean ± 2SD of control value. We also defined the normal protein nutritional state as those who have serum albumin concentrations above 3.5 g/dl [13]. When cirrhotic patients were classified according to the presence or absence of energy malnutrition and protein malnutrition as defined above, 30% of the patients showed protein-energy malnutrition, 40%

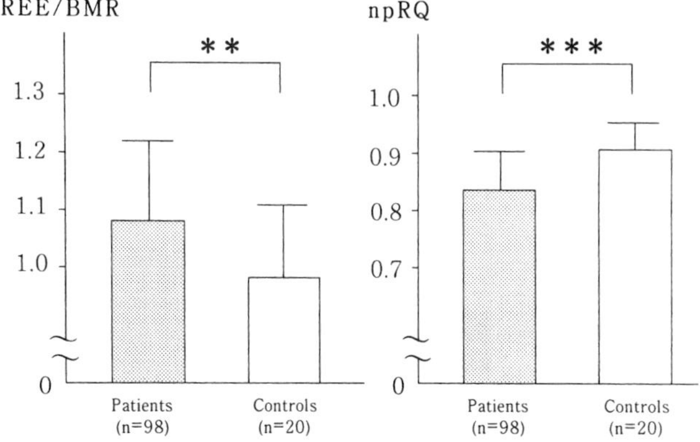

Fig. 1. Resting energy expenditure (REE) standardized by basal metabolic rate (BMR) and nonprotein respiratory quotient (npRQ) in patients with liver cirrhosis and controls. Values are expressed as mean and SD. **$p < 0.01$, ***$p < 0.001$ by the Student's t test.

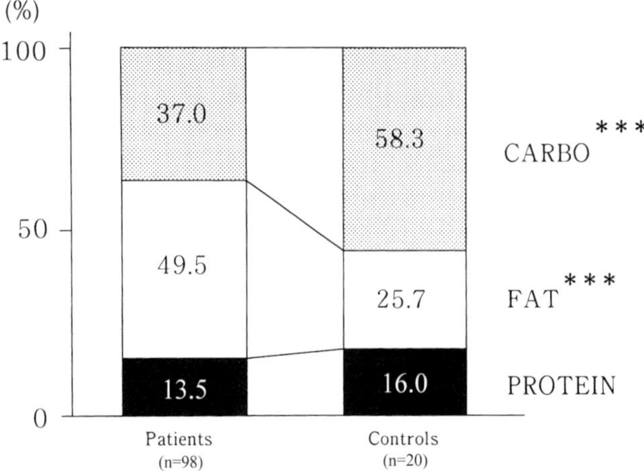

Fig. 2. Oxidation rates of carbohydrate (CARBO), fat (FAT) and protein (PROTEIN) in patients with liver cirrhosis and controls. Values are expressed as mean. ***p < 0.001 by the Student's t test.

showed protein malnutrition alone, 10% showed energy malnutrition alone and the remaining 20% had a normal protein and energy nutritional state (Fig. 5).

Effect of energy metabolism on the survival of cirrhotics

Survival of cirrhotic patients was followed up after calorimetry for up to 7 years. Survival rate estimated by the Kaplan-Meier method was significantly lower in patients with low nonprotein respiratory quotient (npRQ < 0.85, n = 67) than

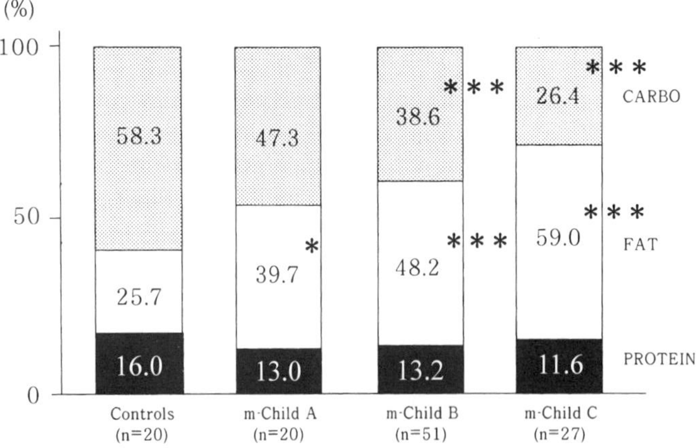

Fig. 3. Oxidation rates of carbohydrate (CARBO), fat (FAT) and protein (PROTEIN) in controls and patients with liver cirrhosis of modified Child's grade A, B or C. Values are expressed as mean. *p < 0.05, ***p < 0.001 as compared with controls by the Dunnett's t test.

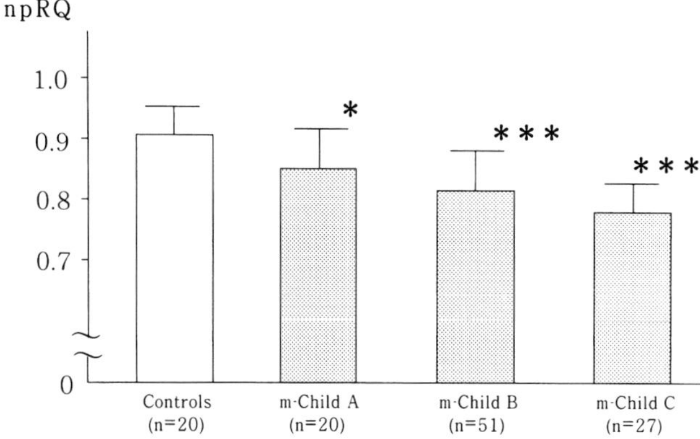

Fig. 4. Nonprotein respiratory quotient (npRQ) in controls and patients with liver cirrhosis of modified Child's grade A, B or C. Values are expressed as mean. *p < 0.05, ***p < 0.001 as compared with controls by the Dunnett's t test.

those with the value above 0.85 (n = 31) (p < 0.05) (Fig. 6). Resting energy expenditure/basal metabolic rate also significantly affected the survival of cirrhotic patients (p < 0.05, curves not shown). Other significant parameters which gave longer survivals were absence of ascites (p < 0.01), serum total bilirubin lower than 2.0 mg/dl (p < 0.01), total protein higher than 7.0 g/dl (p < 0.05), albumin higher than 2.8 g/dl (p < 0.01), plasma hepaplastin test higher than 40% (p < 0.001), prothrombin activity higher than 70% (p < 0.01), blood ammonia below 100 µg/dl (p < 0.01), ICG R15 below 35% (p < 0.01), blood urea nitrogen lower than 10 mg/dl (p < 0.05), serum total cholesterol higher than 150 mg/

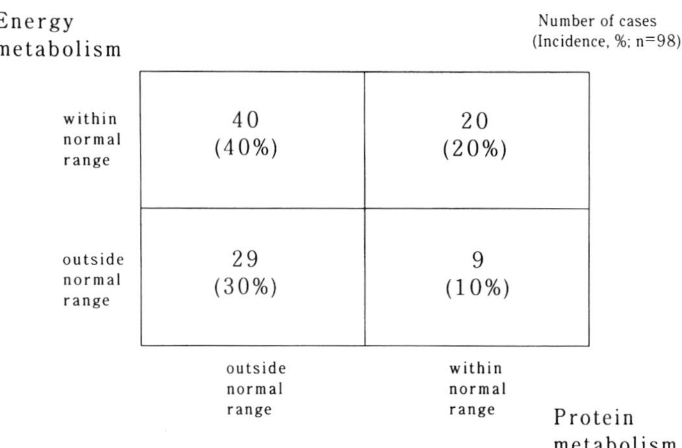

Fig. 5. Number and incidence of subjects with energy or protein malnutrition in cirrhotic patients. For the definition of normal ranges of protein metabolism and energy metabolism, see "Characteristics of energy metabolism in liver cirrhosis" in the text.

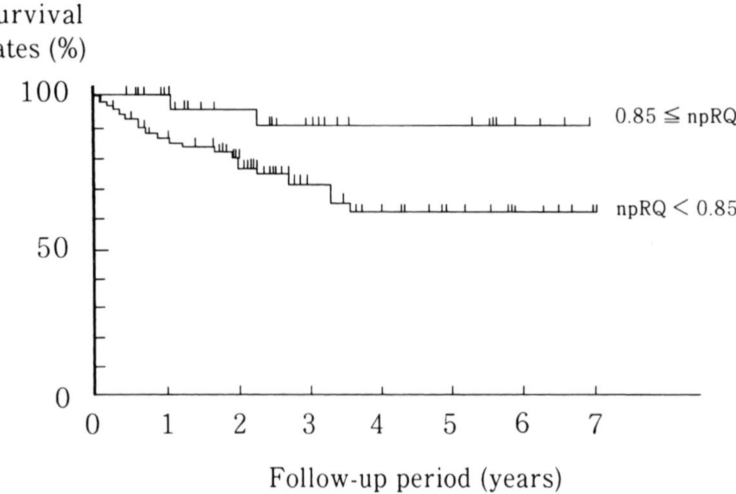

Fig. 6. Kaplan-Meier estimates of the survival in cirrhotic patients with nonprotein respiratory quotient (npRQ) above 0.85 and in those with the value below 0.85. $p < 0.05$ by the log-rank test.

dl ($p < 0.05$), triglyceride higher than 70 mg/dl ($p < 0.05$), and plasma branched chain amino acids/aromatic amino acids molar ratio (Fischer's ratio) above 1.5 ($p < 0.05$).

Such parameters as age, % ideal body weight, % arm muscular circumference, % triceps skin fold, body mass index, serum creatinine, blood lymphocyte count, hemoglobin, platelet count and fasting plasma glucose did not show any significant effect on the survival of cirrhotics. Reliable statistical analysis was not possible regarding the effect of hepatic coma on survival, since hepatic coma appeared only in four patients among 98 cirrhotic subjects in this study.

We then analyzed the survival data by the multivariate proportional hards model. Among significant variables obtained by the univariate analysis as described above, we employed a total of seven parameters of the highest statistical significance. We also limited the number of variables within seven, since the total number of cirrhotics of 98 allowed a maximum number of variables to six or seven for a reliable statistical analysis. These parameters included nonprotein respiratory quotient, resting energy expenditure/basal metabolic rate, presence of ascites, serum total bilirubin and albumin concentrations, plasma hepaplastin test, and blood ammonia concentration. We regarded hepaplastin test and blood ammonia to substitute for prothrombin time and hepatic coma, respectively. Thus, the latter five of the above seven variables are actually the parameters employed in the modified Child's classification [15]. This proportional hazards model analysis demonstrated that serum albumin (relative risk, 0.195, 95% confidence interval, 0.073–0.523), nonprotein respiratory quotient (0.000, 0.000–0.023) and resting energy expenditure (0.007, 0.000–0.531) were

Table 2. Nutritional parameters associated with survival in patients with liver cirrhosis.

Variable	Relative risk	95% Confidence limit		p value
		Lower	Upper	
Albumin	0.195	0.073	0.523	0.0012
npRQ	0.000	0.000	0.023	0.0060
REE/BMR	0.007	0.000	0.531	0.0248

npRQ: nonprotein respiratory quotient; REE: resting energy expenditure; BMR: basal metabolic rate. Variables were eliminated stepwise from ascites, total bilirubin, NH_3, albumin, hepaplastin test, npRQ and REE/BMR using Cox proportional hazards model.

independent significant factors to determine the survival of cirrhotic patients (Table 2).

What is reflected by nutritional parameters of energy metabolism in cirrhotics

Nonprotein respiratory quotient significantly correlated with parameters of functional reserve of the liver such as serum albumin (Fig. 7) and hepaplastin test (r = 0.31, p < 0.01). In addition, significant correlations were also found between nonprotein respiratory quotient and such parameters as total bilirubin (r = −0.32, p < 0.01), prothrombin time (r = 0.30, p < 0.01) and platelet count (r = 0.27, p < 0.01). Nonprotein respiratory quotient did not correlate with anthropometrical parameters or indocyanine green dye clearance. Since a decrease in nonprotein respiratory quotient is determined in part by the reduced glycogen storage and glycogenesis in liver cirrhosis [11], correlations as described above

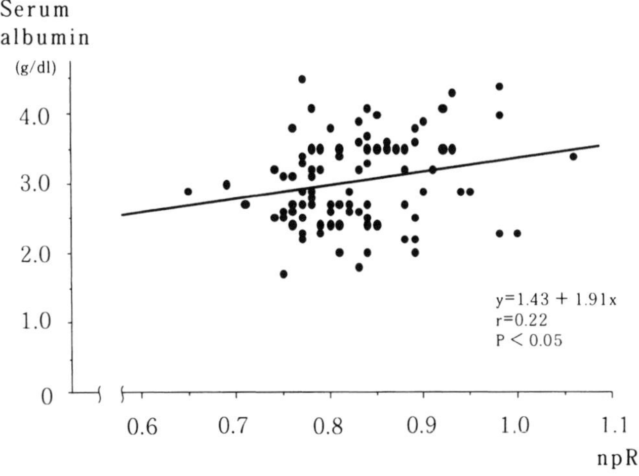

Fig. 7. Significant correlation between nonprotein respiratory quotient (npRQ) and serum albumin in patients with liver cirrhosis.

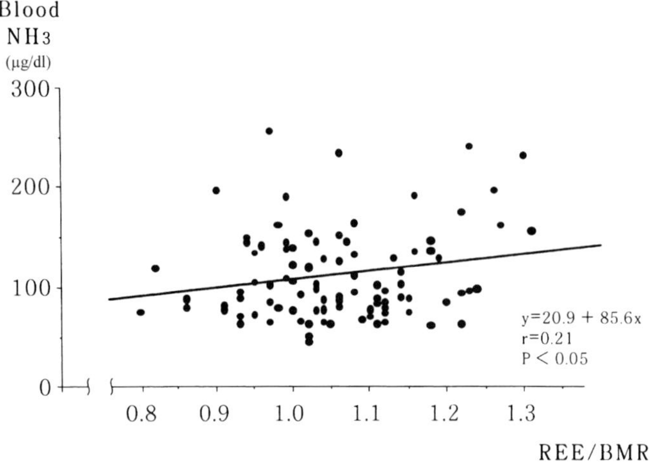

Fig. 8. Significant correlation between resting energy expenditure (REE) standardized by basal metabolic rate (BMR) and blood ammonia (NH$_3$) in patients with liver cirrhosis.

may indicate that nonprotein respiratory quotient reflects largely the hepatic parenchymal function but not the splanchnic blood flow.

Resting energy expenditure significantly correlated only with blood ammonia (Fig. 8) and anthropometrical parameters including body mass index ($r = -0.34$, $p < 0.05$), % triceps skin fold ($r = -0.31$, $p < 0.05$) and % ideal body weight ($r = -0.31$, $p < 0.05$). Blood ammonia level depends on the volume of skeletal muscles in liver cirrhosis [16]. Hence, these correlations may suggest that resting energy expenditure in liver cirrhosis is mainly affected by the body mass composition.

Conclusions

Energy metabolism significantly affects the long-term prognosis of patients with liver cirrhosis. Further investigations are required to elucidate if nutritional support for energy malnutrition improves the survival in these patients.

Acknowledgements

We would like to thank Ms Saori Sugiyama, ward dietician of the department, for her excellent technical assistance to this study.

References

1. Morgan AG, Kelleher J, Walker BE, Losowsky MS. Nutrition in cryptogenic cirrhosis and chronic aggressive hepatitis. Gut 1976;17:113.

2. O'Keefe SJD, El-Zayadi AR, Carraher TE, Davis M, Williams R. Malnutrition and immuno-incompetence in patients with liver disease. Lancet 1980;2:615.

3. Yoshida T, Muto Y, Moriwaki H, Yamato M. Effect of long-term oral supplementation with branched-chain amino acid granules on the prognosis of liver cirrhosis. J Gastroenterol (Gastroenterol Jpn) 1989;24:692.

4. Eriksson LS. Branched-chain amono acids in the treatment of hepatic encephalopathy. In: Conn HO, Bircher J (eds) Hepatic Encephalopathy: Management with Lactulose and Related Carbohydrates. East Lansing, UK: Medi-Ed Press, 1988;129.

5. O'Keefe SJD. Parenteral nutrition and liver disease. In: Rombeau JL, Caldwell MD (eds) Clinical Nutrition-Parenteral Nutrition. Philadelphia: W.B. Saunders, 1993;676.

6. Campillo B, Bories PN, Pornin B, Devanley M. Influence of liver failure, ascites and energy expendiure on the response to oral nutrition in alcoholic liver cirrhosis. Nutrition 1997;13:613.

7. Müller MJ, Böker KH, Selberg O. Metabolism of energy-yielding substrates in patients with liver cirrhosis. Clin Invest 1994;72:568.

8. Müller MJ, Lauts HU, Plogmann B, Burger M, Korber J, Schmidt FW. Energy expenditure and substrate oxidation in patients with cirrhosis: the impact of cause, clinical staging and nutritional state. Hepatology 1992;15:782.

9. Müller MJ, Loyal S, Schwarze M et al. Resting energy expenditure and nutritional state in patients with liver cirrhosis before and 432 days after liver transplantation. Clin Nutr 1994; 13:145.

10. Selberg O, Böttcher J, Tusch G, Pichlmayr R, Henkel E, Müller MJ. Identification of high- or low-risk patients before liver transplantation: a prospective cohort study of nutritional and metabolic parameters in 150 patients. Hepatology 1997;25:652.

11. Kato M, Miwa Y, Tajika M et al. Preferential use of branched-chain amino acids as an energy substrate in patients with liver cirrhosis. Int Med (In press).

12. Konstantinides FN, Boehm KA, Radmer WJ et al. Pyrochemiluminescence: Real time, cost-effective method for determining total urinary nitrogen in clinical nitrogen-balance studies. Clin Chem 1988;34:2518.

13. Harris JA, Benedict FG. A Biometric Study of Basal Metabolism in Man. Washington, DC: Carnegie Institute of Washington, 1919;No. 297.

14. Agarwal NR, Savino JA, Feldman J, Dawson J, Gupte P, Del Guercio LR. The automated metabolic profile. Crit Care Med 1983;11:546.

15. Pugh RNH, Murray-Lyon IM, Dawson JL, Pietroni MS, Williams R. Transection of the oesophagus for bleeding oesophageal varices. Br J Surg 1983;60:646.

16. Hayashi M, Ohnishi H, Kawade Y et al. Augmented utilization of branched-chain amino acids by skeletal muscle in decompensated liver cirrhosis in special relation to ammonia detoxication. J Gastroenterol (Gastroenterol Jpn) 1981;16:64.

Progress in Hepatology, Volume 4.
Liver Cirrhosis Update.
M. Yamanaka et al., editors.

125

Interferon therapy for patients with liver cirrhosis due to hepatitis C virus

Kazuhiko Miyake, Hajime Takikawa and Masami Yamanaka

Department of Medicine, Teikyo University School of Medicine, Tokyo, Japan

Abstract. We treated 31 patients (33–57 years old) with liver cirrhosis due to HCV by IFNα. The total IFN dose and duration was $9,878 \pm 633$ (175–2,403) MU and 14.8 ± 14.6 (3–62) months. The response was defined as complete in cases with normal ALT and negative HCV-RNA at the end and during the post-treatment period of 6 months or more. The rate of a complete response was 20 and 33% in HCV genotype 1b and HCV genotypes 2a and 2b, respectively, and the response rate in patients with low HCV-RNA titers was significantly higher than that with high HCV-RNA titers. A complete response required both total doses of more than 500 MU and therapy duration of more than 15 months. During the average of 44 months after the IFN therapy, hepatocellular carcinomas were detected in 14% of complete responders and in 25% of nonresponders. According to these findings, an IFN treatment regimen recommended to HCV-related cirrhotics is considered to be based on long-term treatment (at least more than 12 months), an intermittent therapy (3 times a week), and a proper IFN dose which can maintain negative serum HCV-RNA for at least 1 year.

Keywords: HCV genotype, hepatitis C virus, hepatocellular carcinoma, interferon therapy, liver cirrhosis.

Introduction

Liver cirrhosis due to hepatitis C virus (HCV) has been documented to be an irreversible end-stage liver disease, the majority of which develops hepatocellular carcinomas as well as liver failure.

Currently, interferon (IFN) is available to eradicate HCV in patients with chronic hepatitis C; approximately 30% of those patients who received IFN therapy successfully eliminated HCV-RNA in Japan [1,2].

IFN is also a good candidate for the treatment of liver cirrhosis with HCV, because a causative therapy for those patients is expected. Since an intensive liver fibrosis is known to be one of the unfavorable predictive factors for IFN treatment of chronic hepatitis C [1,2], it is postulated that it is difficult for liver cirrhosis to have an excellent response to IFN. Regarding the efficacy of IFN to cirrhotic patients, it still remains controversial whether liver cirrhosis with HCV responds well to IFN therapy and what IFN treatment regimen should be selected [3–12].

Address for correspondence: Dr Kazuhiko Miyake, Department of Medicine, Teikyo University School of Medicine, Kaga 2-11-1, Itabashi-ku, Tokyo 173-0003, Japan.

Materials and Methods

Thirty-one patients with histologically proved liver cirrhosis due to HCV were studied with IFN therapy. HCV infection was confirmed by both anti-HCV antibody (third generation, ELISA) and HCV-RNA (Amplicor). The inclusion criteria were:

1) negative HBs Ag,
2) absence of signs of severe liver failure,
3) absence of manifest collateral circulations, and
4) absence of severe thrombocytopenia and/or severe leukocytopenia.

Pretreatment characteristics and IFN therapy of 31 patients who received either IFN-α2a or human lymphoblastoid IFNα are as follows. The male:female ratio was 17:14 and the age was 54.5 ± 8.1 ($33-67$) years old. There were 15 patients with high (10^5 copies/50 μl or more) titers of HCV, and 16 patients with low (less than 10^5 copies/50 μl titers of HCV. There were 25, four and two cases of HCV genotypes 1b, 2a and 2b, respectively. The total administered dose of IFN was 9878 ± 633 ($175-2,403$), and the duration of the therapy was 14.8 ± 14.6 ($3-62$) months.

All patients were observed for more than 6 months after the completion of the treatment. Serum ALT and HCV-RNA levels were monitored every month during the follow-up period. The response to IFN therapy was defined as complete when the ALT was normal and HCV-RNA was negative at the end and during the post-treatment period of 6 months or more. The others were defined as a nonresponse.

The efficacy of IFN therapy was compared between two groups with HCV genotypes 1b and 2a + 2b, and between high- and low-HCV-RNA titers, using the χ^2 method when appropriate. $p < 0.05$ was considered to indicate a significant difference.

Results

Among the 31 cirrhotic patients, the rate of a complete response was 20% in genotype 1b and 33% in genotypes 2a and 2b (no significant difference between HCV genotypes). In contrast, the response rate in patients with low-HCV-RNA titers was significantly higher than that with high-HCV-RNA titers (Table 1).

Figure 1 indicates the effect of total IFN doses and the duration of the therapy on the response in cirrhotic patients. A complete response in cirrhotics required both total doses of more than 500 MU and therapy duration of more than 15 months. Lower doses and shorter duration of the treatment had a lower probability of a complete response.

A representative case of a 38-year-old male with genotype 1b and high viremia (the HCV-RNA level was 10^5 copies/50 μl or more) is shown in Fig. 2. His liver scintigram (Fig. 3) with ^{99m}Tc-phytate was compatible with liver cirrhosis with the atrophic right lobe, the enlarged left lobe and splenomegaly. The first IFN

Table 1. Effect of IFN therapy on cirrhotic patients with HCV.

HCV genotype	Pretreatment HCV-RNA titer	n	Complete responder
1b	high	13	1 (8%)
	low	12	4 (33%)
	total	25	5 (20%)
2a + 2b	high	2	0 (0%)
	low	4	2 (50%)
	total	6	2 (33%)
Total		31	7 (23%)

The response rate in the whole low HCV-RNA group was significantly higher than the whole high HCV-RNA group ($p < 0.05$).

treatment was performed by a standard therapy regimen consisting of daily administration of 9 MU of IFN-α2a for 2 weeks followed by 9 MU IFN-α2a 3 times weekly for 6 months. Serum HCV-RNA became negative 1 month after starting the therapy and remained negative until the end of the therapy. However, his ALT level was elevated and HCV-RNA was reactivated 1 month after the therapy. The second IFN therapy was performed using the same IFN-α2a dose per day. This regimen consisted of daily 12-week administration of IFN followed by 66-week therapy 3 times weekly. In the second therapy, he was treated with a long-term (1.5 year) IFN therapy, and negative HCV-RNA was obtained 1 month after starting the therapy, and was maintained during and after the IFN treatment, resulting in a complete response.

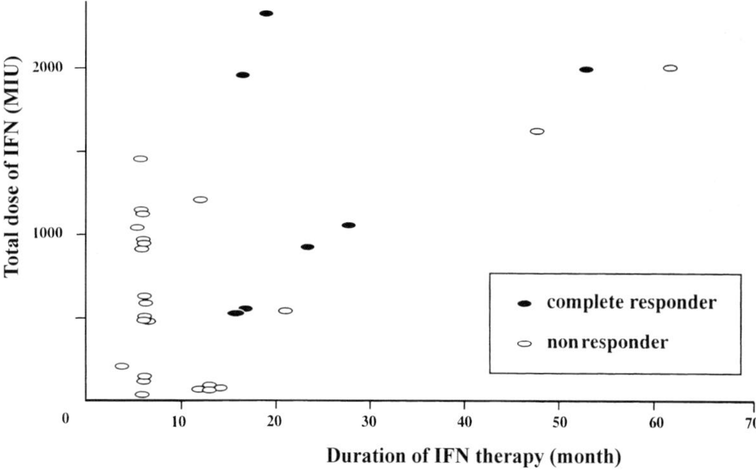

Fig. 1. Relationship between total doses and duration of IFN administered to 31 patients with liver cirrhosis due to HCV.

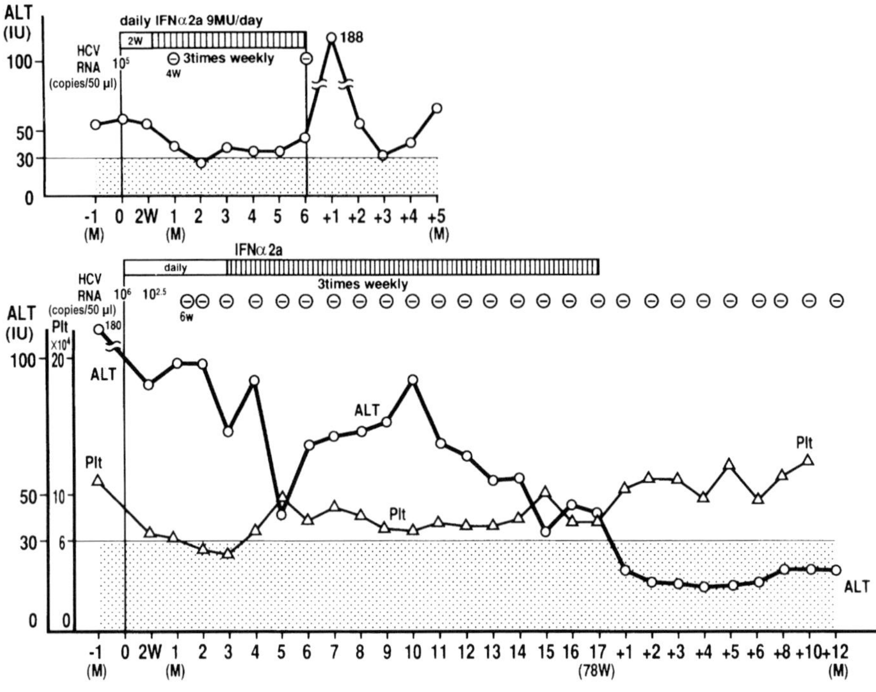

Fig. 2. A representative case of liver cirrhosis with HCV treated with IFN-α2a. The patient was a 38-year-old male and HCV genotype was 1b.

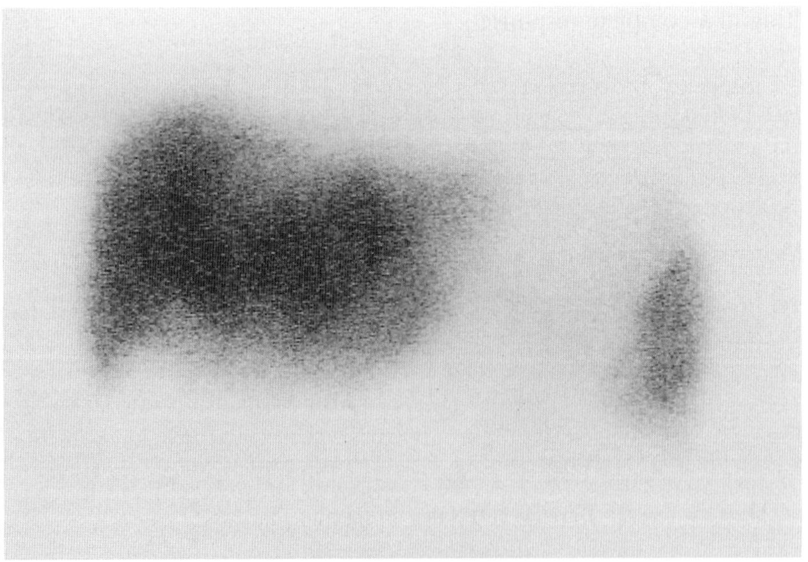

Fig. 3. A liver scintigram with ^{99m}Tc-phytate of the patient presented in Fig. 2.

Table 2 shows the incidence of the appearance of hepatocellular carcinomas and observation periods after the end of the IFN therapy in the cirrhotic patients. The patients were observed in an average of 44 months after the end of the IFN therapy. The development rates of hepatocellular carcinomas were 14% in complete responders and 25% in nonresponders. The difference was not statistically significant. It was 2.5 years after the completion of the IFN therapy that a hepatocellular carcinoma appeared in only one complete responder.

Discussions

The major aim of treating cirrhotic patients with IFN is to prevent the development of hepatocellular carcinomas and progression to liver failure. The response rate to IFN therapy in cirrhotics with HCV is reported to be lower than that in chronic active hepatitis C (Table 3). Complete response rates with IFN therapy are 0–24% in cirrhotics and 15–60% in chronic active hepatitis [3–12]. There are large differences in response rates because of the difference in therapeutic regimens, in the characteristics of the patients including HCV-RNA amounts and genotypes, a large number of quasispecies, and in the duration and the state of the diseases. We summarized the reported results of IFN therapy for chronic active hepatitis and liver cirrhosis due to HCV including those of our present study in Table 4. It clearly reveals the lower efficacy of IFN therapy in cirrhotic patients with the complete response rate of 11 compared to 30% in patients with chronic active hepatitis ($p < 0.05$).

Various host- and HCV-related factors to predict the efficacy of IFN therapy vary in cirrhotic patients and those with chronic active hepatitis. The reasons why the response of IFN therapy in cirrhotics is inferior to the patients without cirrhosis are as follows:
1) the presence of larger numbers of HCV quasispecies in cirrhotics caused by a prolonged duration of HCV infection, making them resistant to IFN therapy,
2) a reduced chance of IFN encountering the receptors of the target-infected hepatocytes because of the disturbance of blood circulation due to intra- and extrahepatic shunt in cirrhotics, and
3) a reduction of numbers of IFN receptors on hepatocytes in cirrhotics.

Our findings failed to show a less-frequent development of hepatocellular carcinomas in complete responders, than in nonresponders with a significant reference due to the small numbers of patients treated (Table 2). Nishiguchi et al. [6]

Table 2. Incidence of the development of hepatocellular carcinomas after IFN therapy in liver cirrhosis with HCV.

Response	n	Incidence of hepatocellular carcinoma	Duration after IFN therapy
Complete responder	7	1 (14%)	45.0 ± 23.3
Nonresponder	24	6 (25%)	43.8 ± 11.7

Table 3. Summary of the reports of IFN therapy for chronic active hepatitis and liver cirrhosis due to HCV.

Author	Year	No. of patients	Diagnosis		Treatment regimen	Duration (months)	Complete response rate	
			CAH	Cirrhosis			CAH (%)	Cirrhosis (%)
Caporaso	1993	81	46	35	3-6MU IFN α2a tiw	12	15	5
Van Thiel	1995	117	22	6	3MU IFN α tiw	6	10	0
			25	6	5MU IFN α tiw	6	17	0
			21	7	3MU IFN α daily	6	19	0
			23	7	5MU IFN α daily	6	32	15
Garson	1995	30	21	9	3MU IFN α tiw	6	19	11
Nishiguchi	1995	45	–	45	6MU IFN α tiw	6	–	16
Puig	1995	34	28	6	3MU IFN α tiw	6	68	17
Pardo	1995	15	–	15	3-6MU IFN α tiw	6	–	0
Van Thiel	1995	31	25	6	5MU IFN α daily or tiw	6	60	0
Picciotto	1995	30	26	4	6MU IFN α tiw	6	55	25
Akahane	1996	67	60	7	6MU IFN α tiw	6	35	14
Ide	1996	61	29	–	6MU IFN α daily 2w + tiw 14-16w	6	31	–
			–	32	3-6MU IFN α daily 1-2w + tiw 22-23w	6	–	16
Present study		31	–	31	3-9MU IFN α daily 2-12w + tiw ≥ 26w	6	–	23

Data are adopted from [3–12]. CAH, chronic active hepatitis; tiw, 3 times a week.

reported that IFN treatment reduced the risk of hepatocellular carcinomas in patients with HCV-associated liver cirrhosis. Therefore, IFN therapy will prevent hepatocellular carcinomas in patients with liver cirrhosis if they are treated at an early a stage of cirrhosis as possible.

IFN regimen for liver cirrhosis with HCV is basically similar to that for chronic hepatitis C. The inclusion criteria for the IFN treatment of cirrhotics are:
1) abnormal ALT levels,
2) absence of hepatitis B surface antigen and other potential causes of chronic liver diseases,
3) absence of manifest collateral circulations,

Table 4. Summary of reported results of IFN therapy for patients with chronic active hepatitis and liver cirrhosis due to HCV.

Diagnosis	No. of patients	Complete response rate (%) (HCV clearance)
Chronic active hepatitis	326	30[a]
Liver cirrhosis	216	11[a]

Data are adopted from [3–12] (Table 3). [a]p < 0.05.

4) compensated cirrhosis, and

5) platelet counts $> 10 \times 10^4$ and leukocyte counts $> 4,000$ in the peripheral blood.

A favorable IFN treatment regimen for cirrhotics is based on

1) long-term treatment (at least more than 12 months),

2) an intermittent therapy (3 times a week), and

3) a proper IFN dose per day which can maintain negative serum HCV-RNA for at least 1 year during IFN therapy.

We also need to pay a lot of attention to autoimmune disorders and bacterial infection in cases of severe leukocytopenia as well as an occurrence of psychological disturbances, particularly anxiety-depression and schizophrenia.

We can have a more favorable efficacy of IFN therapy for patients with liver cirrhosis due to HCV, who have never been cured with other agents. Further progress in therapeutic regimens is needed to obtain better results.

References

1. Tsubota A, Chayama K, Ikeda K, Arase Y, Koida I, Saitoh S, Hashimoto M, Iwasaki S, Kobayashi M, Kumada H. Factors predictive of response to interferon alpha therapy in hepatitis C virus infection. Hepatology 1994;19:1088–1094.
2. Hayashi J, Ohmiya M, Kishihara Y, Yoshiki T, Minukawa N, Ikematsu H, Kashiwagi S. A statistical analysis of predictive factors of response to human lymphoblastoid interferon in patients with chronic hepatitis C. Am J Gastroenterol 1994;89:2151–2156.
3. Caporaso N, Suozzo R, Marisco F, D'Antonio M, Romano M. Recombinant human interferon alpha-2a therapy for chronic hepatitis C with or without cirrhosis. Ital J Gastroenterol 1993; 25:482–486.
4. Van Thiel DH, Friedlander L, Fagivoli S, Malloy PJ, Kania RJ. The Oklahoma-Pittsburgh experience with interferon-α in the treatment of HCV disease. J Oklahoma State Med Assoc 1995;88:4.
5. Garson JA, Brillanti S, Whitby K, Foli M, Deaveille R. Analysis of clinical and virological factors associated with response to alpha interferon therapy in chronic hepatitis C. J Med Virol 1995;45:348–353.
6. Nishiguchi S, Kuroki T, Nakatani S, Morimoto H, Takeda T. Randomised trial of effects of interferon-α on incidence of hepatocellular carcinoma in chronic active hepatitis C with cirrhosis. Lancet 1995;346:1051–1055.
7. Puig P, Dussaix E, Altman C, Lavel C, Stuyver L. Host and viral characteristics affecting the response to interferon therapy in chronic hepatitis C. Eur J Gastroenterol Hepatol 1995;7: 335–340.
8. Pardo M, Castillo I, Navas S, Carreno V. Treatment of chronic hepatitis C with cirrhosis with recombinant human granulocyte colony stimulating factor plus recombinant interferon-α. J Med Virol 1995;45:439–444.
9. Van Thiel DH, Friedlander L, Fagiuoli S, Molloy PJ, Kania RJ. Interferon alpha can be used successfully in patients with hepatitis C virus positive chronic hepatitis who have a psychiatric illness. Eur J Gastroenterol Hepatol 1995;7:165–168.
10. Picciotto A, Callea F, Varagona G, Bardellini E, Borzone S. Lymphoblastoid interferon therapy in chronic hepatitis C. Liver 1995;15:20–24.
11. Akahane Y, Miyazaki Y, Naitoh S, Takeda K, Tsuda F. Cold activation of complement for monitoring the response to interferon in patients with chronic hepatitis C. Am J Gastroenterol 1996; 91:319–327.

12. Ide T, Sata M, Suzuki H, Murashima S, Miyajima I, Shirachi M, Tanikawa K. Evaluation of interferon treatment in cirrhotic patients with hepatitis C. J Jpn Assoc Infect Dis 1996;70: 597—604.

Progress in Hepatology, Volume 4.
Liver Cirrhosis Update.
M. Yamanaka et al., editors.

133

Progress in bioartificial liver support

Ikuo Nagashima[1], Katsutoshi Naruse[2], Yasuyuki Sakai[3], Tetsuichiro Muto[2] and Kota Okinaga[1]

[1]*Department of Surgery II, Teikyo University School of Medicine, Tokyo;* [2]*Department of Surgery, Faculty of Medicine, University of Tokyo, Tokyo; and* [3]*Institute of Industrial Science, University of Tokyo, Tokyo, Japan*

Abstract. The evolution of bioartificial liver support system has accelerated in the last decade. At last, some bioartificial livers with hollow fiber (HF) cartridge systems, culturing hepatocytes within the cartridge are being employed, and clinical evaluations of this bioartificial liver has begun. However, it still remains to be seen whether these bioreactors show sufficient hepatic function qualitatively or quantitatively, because no follow-up cases have been reported since their first clinical reports.

We are presenting a new bioreactor with nonwoven polyester fabric (NWF), which is known to be a good fabric for attachment of cultured cells. Our NWF system secretes far more albumin per day than the HF cartridge system, which may be due to the high capacity of hepatocyte cells and mass transfer. In addition, extracorporeal hemoperfusion using the NWF bioreactor significantly prolongs the survival time of pigs suffering from hepatic failure, with the improvement of some values of blood chemistry.

Keywords: bioartificial liver, hepatic failure, nonwoven fabric.

Introduction

Although orthotopic liver transplantation has been an essential treatment for acute and chronic liver failure, the need for a liver assist device still exists. Transplantation is often delayed for technical or medical reasons, and temporary liver support may be life sustaining during this period. Furthermore, some acute and reversible forms of liver failure, such as those resulting from drug overdose and viral hepatitis, have the potential for regeneration and recovery if short-term liver support is provided.

The development of an artificial liver has been a significant challenge. Many early artificial liver techniques failed due to inadequate support of multiple essential hepatic functions, including gluconeogenesis, synthesis of blood protein, amino acid metabolism, urea synthesis, lipid metabolism, drug biotransformation, and waste removal. Overall, about 70% of the patients showed neurologic improvement, however, only 28% survived after treatment [1].

In these situations, a bioartificial liver comprising viable hepatocytes on a mechanical support so-called hybrid liver support system, has been considered

Address for correspondence: Ikuo Nagashimam MD, Department of Surgery II, Teikyo University School of Medicine, 2-11-1 Kaga, Itabashi-ku, Tokyo 173-8605, Japan.

134

to be more likely to provide these essential functions than a purely mechanical device [2].

In this paper, we review the evolution of bioartificial liver support during the last decade. Both historical and state-of-the-art techniques are discussed. Also, we show our new technique of a nonwoven polyester fabric (NWF) bioreactor for the progress of bioartificial liver support system.

Current evolution of bioartificial liver systems

Based on the limited success achieved using early liver support techniques [3], the concept evolved so that liver functions essential for survival would be best provided by mammalian liver preparations [2]. These liver preparations, commonly referred to as hybrid or bioartificial systems, contain biologic components within a synthetic framework. Biologic components may include isolated liver enzymes [4—7], cellular components [7,8], slices of liver [9,10], or cultured hepatocytes [11,12].

Of all of them, hepatocyte systems have shown the greatest promise for bioartificial liver support. Hepatocyte systems supplied a greater number of liver functions, since they utilize intact, metabolically active liver cells [13]. Hepatocyte systems may be implanted in the patents [11] or perfused extracorporeally [12]. However, drawbacks of implantable hepatocyte systems have been identified [2]. Thus, extracorporeal bioartificial liver designs offer on-line artificial liver support.

In general, these medical devices are designed for short-term support of medical therapy, or as a bridge to liver transplantation. Of several extracorporeal bioartificial systems, two extracorporeal systems that have undergone extensive testing are hepatocyte suspension systems [12] and hollow fiber (HF) cartridge systems [13,14]. Suspension cultures are easily scaled up; however, hepatocytes are anchorage-dependent and rapidly loose viability and function in suspension culture.

On the other hand, hepatocyte viability and function are improved in adhesion culture [15], although surface area and cell attachment become limitations to scale-up. Since HF cartridges offer a large surface area for mass transport, the HF cartridge system is employed as a bioartificial liver, culturing hepatocytes within the cartridge. Clinical evaluations of this bioartificial liver configuration with HF system have begun [16—18]. It has been reported that significant clinical improvements occurred in several patients with hepatic failure; however, no follow-up cases have been reported.

Development of a bioartifical liver support system with the NWF bioreactor

Hepatocyte viability and function are difficult to maintain at the high cell density required in a bioartificial liver. With this difficulty in mind, many designs utilize HF cartridges in order to enhance nutrient transport to the cultured cells. However, the bioartificial liver must fulfill certain biologic requirements in order to support a viable, functioning hepatocyte cell mass. Here, we took up NWF which is known to be a good fabric for attachment of cultured cells [19,20] as a material to immobilize large amounts of cultured hepatocytes in a bioreactor.

Preparation of a NWF column

NWF sheet (150 × 270 × 4 mm; Chiyoda Corporation, Japan) was soaked and agitated overnight in CCL4 solution, washed in ethanol, rinsed with water, then soaked overnight in 0.03% collagen solution (Gibco) to achieve coating with collagen, and allowed to dry. This NWF sheet was wound around the shaft and tightly packed into a 200-ml polycarbonate column, which was then sterilized with ethylene-oxide gas. Thereafter, the NWF column with a radial-flow design, in which afferent blood initially diffuses to the periphery and then returns to the center through the packed NWF, was prepared (Fig. 1).

Porcine hepatocyte isolation

The Sangen-strain pig weighing 10—15 kg underwent the operation as follows to take isolated hepatocytes. The portal vein was catheterized, and 2,000 ml of physiological saline with 2,000 units of heparin were infused with the pressure of 200 cmH$_2$O. Instantly, the hepatoduodenal ligament excluding the portal vein was ligated and divided. The inferior vena cava was also divided for liver dehematization. Then the whole liver was resected and placed on the back table, and the inferior vena cava was catheterized to complete the perfusion circuit. Hepatocytes were then isolated by Seglen's method as follows [21]. First, Hanks-HEPES buffer (37°C) supplemented with 2.0 mM of EDTA (ethylene-diamine tetoraacetic acid) and 1.0 mM of EDTA (ethylene-glycol tetoraacetic acid) was perfused for 15 min at a rate of 200 ml/min. Then, 0.05% collagenase solution (37°C) was perfused for 30 min at the same rate. The capsule of liver was torn and the isolated hepatocytes were dispersed into 0.05% collagenase solution. This crude hepatocyte solution underwent several cycles of pipetting, centifiguration at 660 rpm (50 g) and purification using Eagle's medium (MEM) (4°C). Thereafter, genuine isolated hepatocytes were obtained.

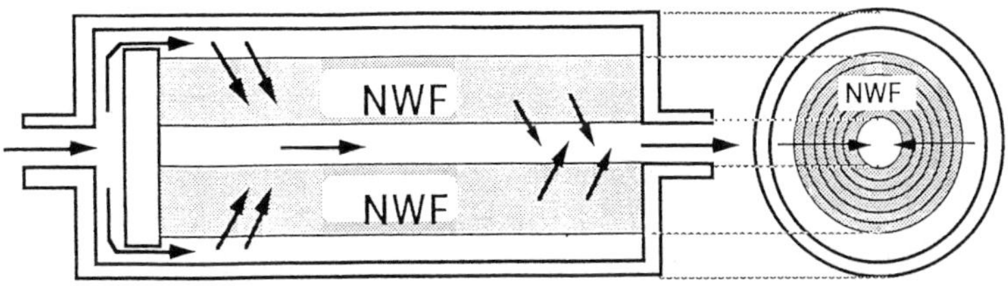

Fig. 1. Diagram of the 200-ml NWF bioreactor with a radial-flow design.

Hepatocyte immobilization in the NWF bioreactor

Isolated hepatocyte solution containing 1.0×10^{10} cells was initially placed in a 1 l reservoir bottle equipped with a DO valve, and suspended with William's Eagle (WE) medium supplemented with 10% fetal bovine serum, 10^{-8} M insulin, 10^{-7} M dexamethasone, 100 units/ml penicillin and 1.0 Ug/ml amphotericin B. The reservoir containing hepatocytes, the 200-ml NWF column and a roller pump were connected in this order with silicon tubes to complete the perfusion circuit. Perfusion was begun at a rate of 30 ml/min, and the hepatocytes were trapped in the NWF column for the next 24 h. Oxygen was supplied to the reservoir bottle through a silicon tube wound around the shaft of the stirrer bar. The DO valve was maintained at 6.0–8.0 ppm by introducing highly pressured (1 kgf/cm^2) 95% O_2/5% CO_2 into the tubing. An electron microscopic photograph of the hepatocytes immobilized or trapped in the network of NWFs is shown in Fig. 2. In addition, the 200-ml NWF reactor showed 0.625 mM/h ammonia removal and 0.706 mM/h urea synthesis over 2 h. It also secreted 3.57 g/day of albumin, which is far superior to the data of the HF bioreactor in the study by Nyberg et al. [22,23] (Table 1).

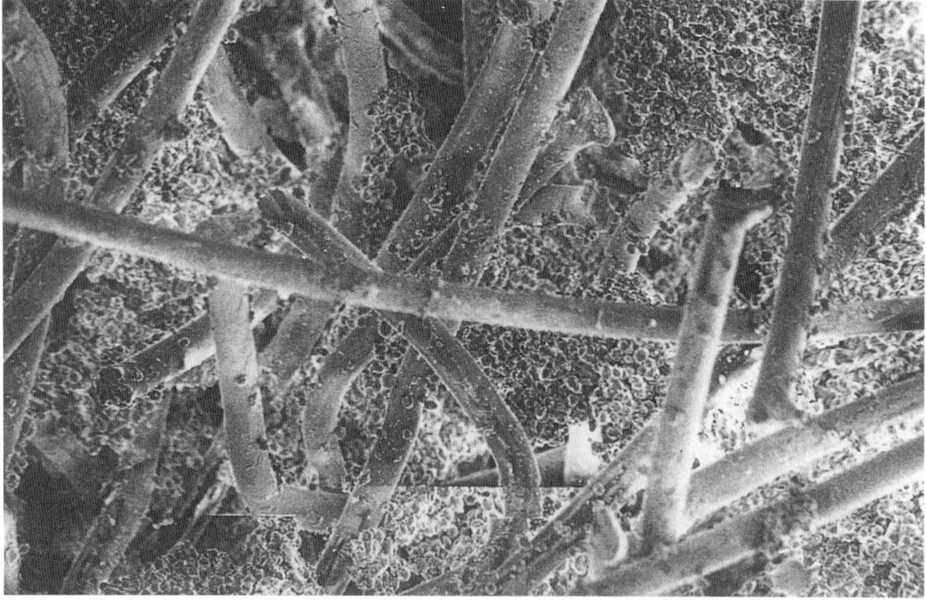

Fig. 2. An electron microscopic photograph of hepatocytes immobilized in the NWF bioreactor.

Table 1. Comparison of efficacy between a NWF bioreactor and a HF bioreactor.

	Cell No. (/bioreactor)	Ammonia removal (mM/h)	Urea synthesis (mM/h)	Albumin secretion (g/day)
NWF	1×10^{10}	0.32	0.42	3.6
HF	1×10^{8}	—	0.28	0.00061
(Nyberg et al. [23])				

Extracorporeal hemoperfusion with the NWF bioreactor for acute hepatic failure in pig — experimental study

Production of hepatic failure model of pig

The Sagen-strain pigs weighing 10–15 kg underwent portal vein and hepatic artery ligation and side-to-side portocaval shunting. These pigs were divided into three groups as follows:
1) control (cont) group (n = 4): no extracorporeal hemoperfusion,
2) column (col) group (n = 4): extracorporeal hemoperfusion using the NWF column without hepatocytes, and
3) bioreactor (bio) group (n = 4): extracorporeal hemoperfusion with the NWF bioreactor.

Extracorporeal hemoperfusion

Four hours later, the operation inducing hepatic failure, pigs of the col and bio group underwent 1 h of extracorporeal hemoperfusion at a flow rate of 30 ml/ min (Fig. 3). The col group was connected with the pure NWF column without hepatocytes, while the bio group with the NWF bioreactor was prepared as mentioned above.

Survival time

The mean survival times of cont, col, and bio groups were 28.0, 26.7, and 35.7 h, respectively, after the operation inducing hepatic failure. The bio group survived significantly longer than each of the others.

Blood chemistry

Blood samples were taken from all pigs before, and just after, the operation inducing hepatic failure (time = 0); just before (time = 4) and after (time = 5) the extracorporeal hemoperfusion; and at 10 h after the operation inducing hepatic failure (time = 10; this meant 5 h after the completion of extracorporeal hemoperfusion). Statistical analysis was performed with ANOVA-method.

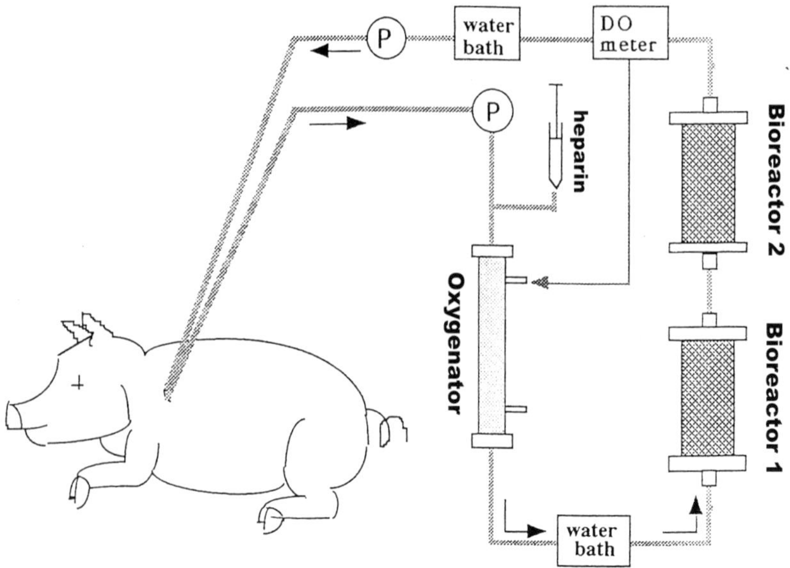

Fig. 3. Schematic representation of extracorporeal hemoperfusion by the NWF bioreactor for acute hepatic failure in pig.

Ammonia (Fig. 4A). The serum ammonia level of the bio group significantly decreased after extracorporeal hemoperfusion compared with that of before hemoperfusion (p = 0.013), while that of either the cont group or the col group increased gradually. In addition, the serum ammonia level of the bio group was significantly lower than that of either the cont group or the col group 10 h after the operation inducing hepatic failure (p = 0.038).

Total bile acid (Fig. 4B). The serum total bile acid level of the bio group significantly decreased after extracorporeal hemoperfusion compared with that of before the hemoperfusion (p = 0.026), while that of the cont group increased gradually. In addition, the serum total bile acid level of the bio group was significantly lower than that of either the cont group or the col group 10 h after the operation inducing hepatic failure (p = 0.040).

Glucose (Fig. 4C). The serum glucose level of the bio group significantly increased after extracorporeal hemoperfusion compared with that of before the hemoperfusion (p = 0.026), while that of either the cont group or col group decreased gradually. In addition, the serum glucose level of the bio group was significantly higher than that of either the cont group or the col group 10 h after the operation inducing hepatic failure (p = 0.045).

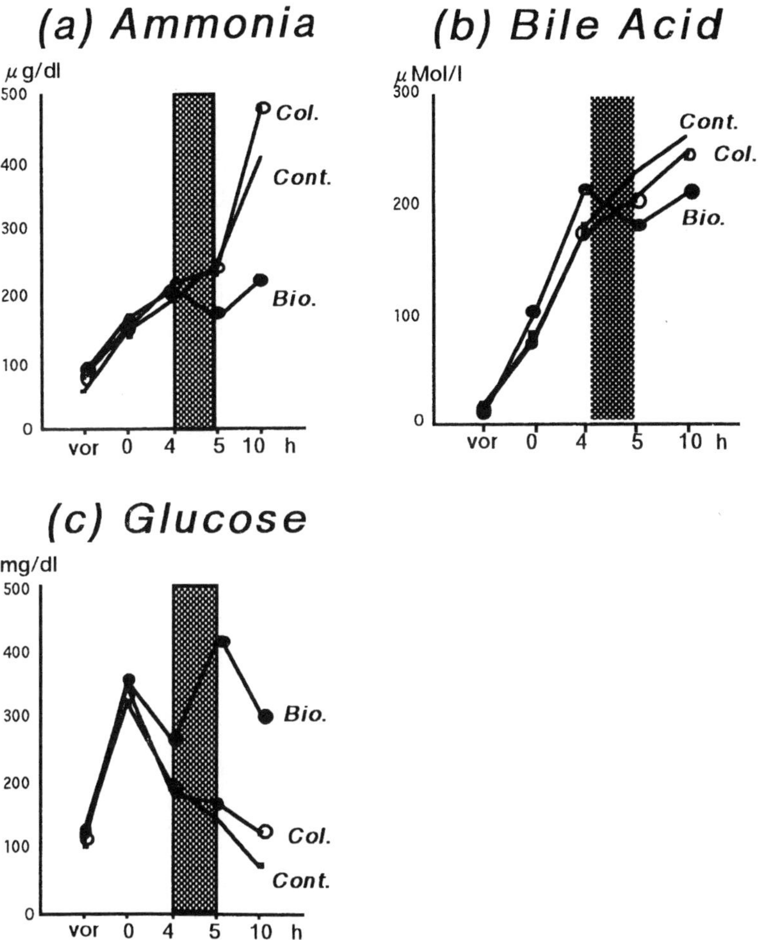

Fig. 4. Changes of mean values of blood chemistry in pigs with acute hepatic failure, up to each group as follows: cont: •, col: ○, and bio: ⬤; (a): ammonia, (b): total bile acid, (c): glucose.

Conclusion

Extracorporeal hemoperfusion using the NWF bioreactor significantly prolonged the survival time of pigs which suffered from liver failure. In addition, the values of blood chemistry indicated that some hepatic functions were significantly improved after extracorporeal hemoperfusion.

Discussion

In this last decade, the bioartificial liver, especially utilizing HF cartridge immobilized mammalian hepatocytes, has been proposed and developed evolutionally.

Some clinical trials for acute or chronic hepatic failure that demonstrated beneficial effect from extracorporeal hemoperfusion using the bioartificial liver with HF cartridge system, have been reported [16–18]. Although those clinical reports were so attractive, we regret that neither follow-up case studies nor randomized trials have been reported since then. It still remains to be seen whether these bioreactors utilizing HF cartridge show sufficient hepatic function qualitatively or quantitatively.

We presented a new bioreactor with NWF, which is known to be a good fabric for attachment of cultured cells. Our NWF system secreted far more albumin per day than the HF cartridge system, which may be due to the high capacity of hepatocyte cells and mass transfer [22,23]. In addition, extracorporeal hemoperfusion using the NWF bioreactor significantly prolonged the survival time of pigs suffering from hepatic failure, with improvement of some blood chemistry values. Although the NWF system for bioartificial liver may make a significant contribution to the development of a hybrid artificial liver system, our study is preliminary and ongoing. Further study should be required.

References

1. Nybergs SL, Peshwa MV, Payne WD, Hu WS, Cerra FB. Evolution of the bioartificial liver: the need for randomized clinical trials. Am J Surg 1993;166:512–521.
2. Jauregui HO, Gann KL. Mammalian hepatocytes as a foundation for treatment in human liver failure. J Cell Biochem 1991;45:359–365.
3. Takahashi T, Malchesky PS, Nose Y. Artificial liver: state of the art. Dig Dis Sci 1991;36:1327–1340.
4. Brunner G, Tegtmeier F. Enzymatic detoxification using lipophilic hollow-fiber membranes: I. Glucuronidation reactions. Artif Organs 1984;8:161–166.
5. Tegtmeier F, Brunner G. Enzymatic detoxification using lipophilic hollow-fiber membranes: II. Sulfation reactions. Artif Organs 1985;9:37–41.
6. Lavin A, Sung C, Klibanov AM, Langer A. Enzymatic removal of bilirubin from blood: a potential treatment for neonatal jaundice. Science 1985;230:543–545.
7. Chang TM. Experimental artificial liver support with emphasis of fulminant hepatic failure: concepts and review. Sem Liv Dis 1986;6:148–158.
8. Yamamoto Y, Tsikas D, Brunner G. Enzymatic detoxification using lipophilic hollow-fiber membranes: III. Oxidation reactions of sulfides. Artif Organs 1989;13:103–108.
9. Koshino I, Sakamoto H, Shinada Y et al. Use of liver slices for: artificial liver. Trans ASAIO 1979;25:493–496.
10. Lie TS, Jung V, Kachel F, Hohnke C, Lee KS. Successful treatment of hepatic coma by a new artificial liver device in the pigs. Res Exp Med (Berl) 1985;185:483–494.
11. Demetriou AA, Whiting JF, Feldman D et al. Replacement of a liver function in ruts by transplantation of microcarrier-attached hepatocytes. Science 1986;233:1190–1192.
12. Matsumuru KN, Guevara GA, Huston H et al. Hybrid bioartificial liver in hepatic failure: preliminary clinical report. Surgery 1987;101:99–103.
13. Hager JC, Carmen A, Porter LE et al. Neonatal hepatocyte culture on artificial capillaries: a model for drug metabolism and the artificial liver. ASAIO J 1983;6:26–35.
14. Demetriou AA, Whiting J, Levenson SM et al. New method of hepatocyte transplantation and extracorporeal liver support. Ann Surg 1986;204:259–271.
15. Gerlach J, Kloppel K, Schauwecker HH, Tauber A, Muuler C, Bucherl ES. Use of hepatocyte in

adhesion and suspension cultures for liver support bioreactors. Int J Artif Organs 1989;12: 788—792.

16. Rozga J, Holzmun MD, Ro MS et al. Development of a hybrid bioartificial liver. Ann Surg 1993;217:502—511.

17. Neizil DF, Rozga J, Mossioni AD et al. Use of a novel bioartificial liver in a patient with acute liver insufficiency. Surgery 1993;13:340—343.

18. Sussman NL, Kelly JH. Improved liver function following treatment with an extracorporeal liver assist device. Artif Organs 1993;17:27—30.

19. Mitsuda S, Matsuda Y, Itagaki Y et al. Nonwoven fabrics as a new cell matrices for IMR-90 human embryonic lung diploid fibroblast cells. J Ferment Bioeng 1990;70:289—291.

20. Matsumura M, Motobu M, Matsuo S, Yamazaki Y, Kataoka H. Bioreactor with a radial-flow nonwoven fabric bed form animal cell culture. Anim Cell Tech. Basic & Applied. Dordrecht: Kluwer Acad Pub, 1993:433—442.

21. Seglen PO. Preparation of isolated liver cells. Method in Cell Biology, Vol 13. In: Prescott DM (ed) New York: Academic Press, 1976:29—83.

22. Naruse K, Sakai Y, Nagashima I, Jiang GX, Suzuki M, Muto T. Development of a new bioartificial liver module filled with porcine hepatocytes immobilized on nonwoven fabric. Int J Artif Organs 1996;6:347—352.

23. Nyberg SL, Shatford RA, Peshwa MV, White JG, Cerra FB, Hu WS. Evaluation of a hepatocyte-entrapment hollow fiber bioreactor: a potential bioartificial liver. Biotech Bioeng 1993;41: 194—203.

Index of authors

Keyword index